HERBALISM AT HOME

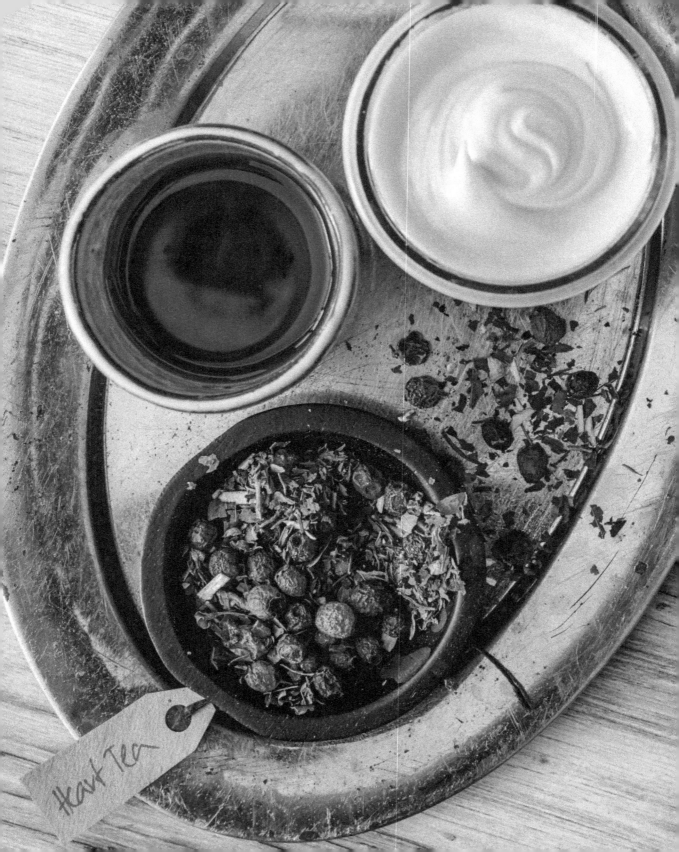

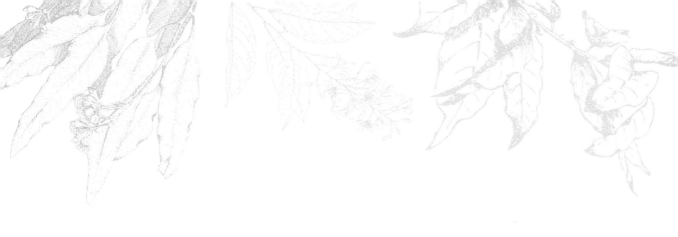

HERBALISM
at home

125 RECIPES
for everyday health

KRISTINE BROWN, RH (AHG)

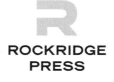

**ROCKRIDGE
PRESS**

Interior and Cover Designer: Linda Snorina
Art Producer: Karen Williams
Editor: Vanessa Ta
Production Manager: Riley Hoffman
Production Editor: Melissa Edeburn

Author photo courtesy of Andrew Dobson

Photography © Evi Abeler

Food styling by Albane Sharrard, cover and pp. ii, vi, x, 74, 76, 106, 120, 144, 160, 172, 198, 222; © Helene Dujardin pp. 19, 21, 36, 41; © Marija Vidal p. 47 (Calendula); Istock, pp. 14, 15, 16, 20, 22, 23, 24, 25, 26, 27, 28, 30, 32, 33, 34, 37, 38, 39, 40, 42, 43, 44, 45, 46, 48, 49, 50 (Passion Flower), 51, 53; Shutterstock, pp. 17, 18, 29, 47 (Cleavers), 50 (New England Aster), 52.

Illustration © Tom Bingham

ISBN: Print 978-1-64611-156-5 | Ebook 978-1-64611-157-2

R0

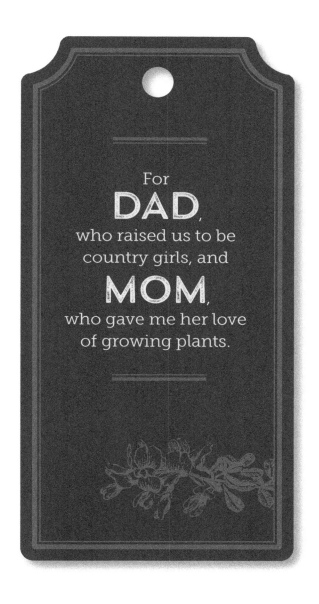

For
DAD,
who raised us to be
country girls, and

MOM,

who gave me her love
of growing plants.

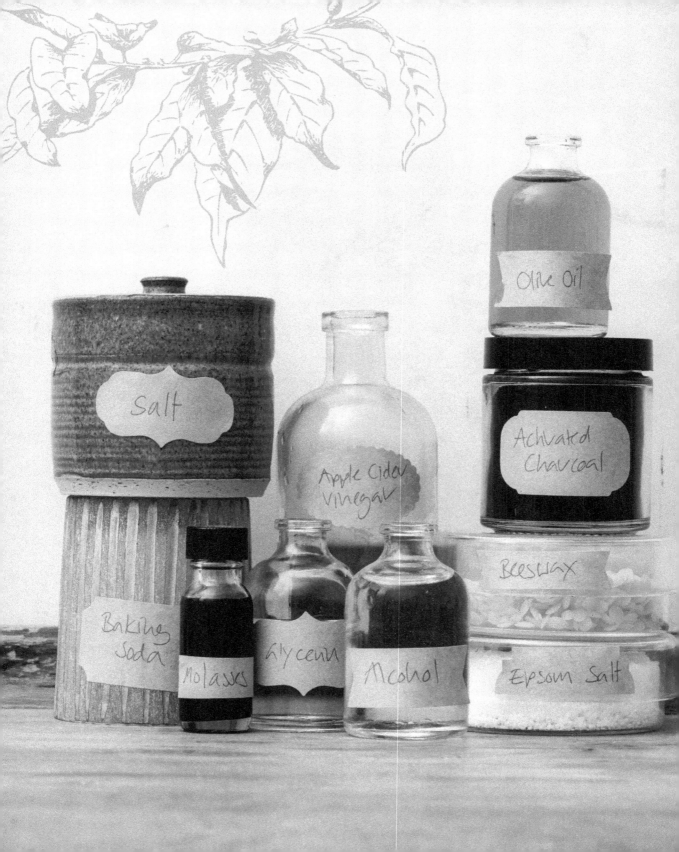

CONTENTS

INTRODUCTION

Growing up, I was fortunate enough to live in the country with access to the woods, a pond, and a pony to ride wherever I wanted to enjoy the sounds and sights of nature.

I also spent many weekends with my paternal grandmother, listening to stories of her many uses of the plants that grew in her yard, both cultivated and weedy.

My journey into herbalism began when I began raising a family of my own. I wanted my children to be healthy, and the more I learned about the toxicity of chemicals and commercial pharmaceuticals, the more I began to notice their overuse.

At one point, my daughter had a swollen lymph node but presented no signs of illness. I took her to the doctor, who immediately prescribed antibiotics and wasn't happy when I questioned the need for them. I picked up the prescription but didn't use it. Instead, I made a weak poke root tea and gave my daughter a small cup of it to drink. The next day, her lymph node was completely back to normal, and she never had another problem with it.

Another time, my older children brought home pertussis (whooping cough) from school. They had been vaccinated against the highly contagious illness, but my younger children had not, and most of us came down with it. The doctor prescribed an antibiotic, which turned out not only to be unnecessary for one of my children (her test came back showing the bacteria had died off), but also to be the *wrong* antibiotic. I immediately switched to an all-herbal protocol for myself and my other kids to calm the intense coughing spasms at night. The herbs soothed our coughs and helped us sleep during that miserable time.

If you're like me, you probably have a relatable story or two about how the medical system has let you down, and that experience might be what led you to pick up this book. Now more than ever, with our health system in crisis, natural health and herbalism are gaining popularity. Medical care costs are on the rise, the quality is questionable, and many people want more natural options that don't come with horrible side effects. At the same time, resources for good, quality herbs also are on the rise, as is good information on how to use them.

Figuring out which of the world's thousands upon thousands of herbs to use can be daunting. In the following chapters, I've helped narrow down the choices by selecting herbs and creating recipes for a variety of common ailments for adults and children, men and women, young and old. These simple, affordable remedies are effective and can be easily made at home. Although this book doesn't cover serious long-term illnesses (consult a qualified herbalist to work out an individual protocol for your specific needs), it does show you how to make your own teas, tinctures, and salves for everyday healing.

This book presents the basics of herbal preparations, along with 40 herb profiles, 125 recipes, tool and ingredient lists, a glossary of herbal terms, and a resource section to help you source reliable information and learn more about herbalism.

Ready to get started? Grab yourself a cup of tea, find a cozy spot to sit, and start reading!

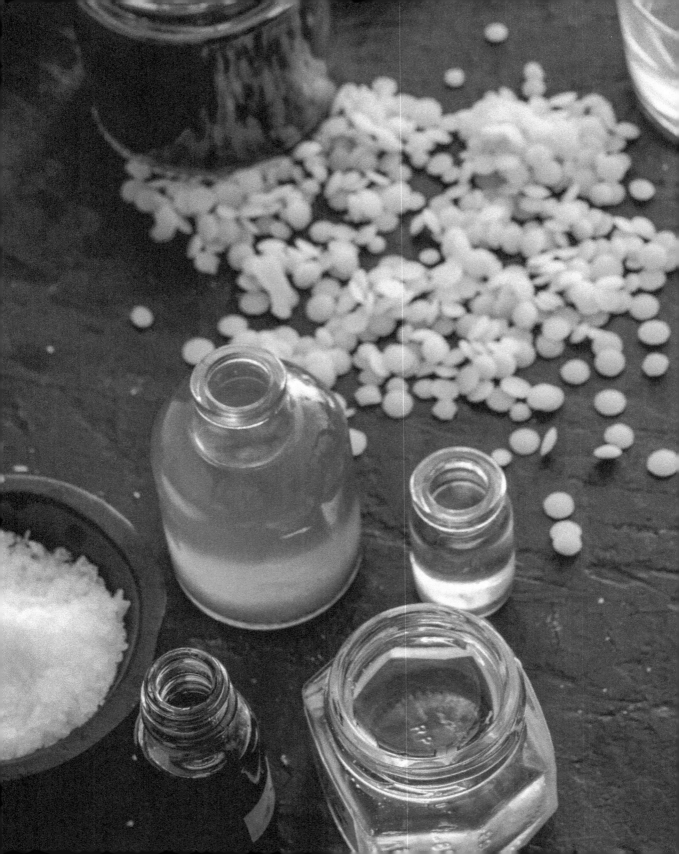

PART ONE

WHAT TO KNOW ABOUT HERBALISM

More and more people are turning to herbalism to provide for their everyday health needs and for good reason—herbs work! If you're new to herbalism, the choices can be daunting. Moreover, most herbs don't come in a box with instructions for how to use them.

What is herbalism? How do you know what to do and when? What are tinctures, teas, infusions, tonics, and salves? How do you make them?

In part 1, I'll answer all these and other questions.

CHAPTER ONE
HERBALISM

In this chapter, we'll explore the history of herbalism, how our ideas about using plants have changed over time, and the benefits of practicing herbalism at home. Confused about when to use conventional medicine rather than herbalism? This chapter will help you make that determination.

By the end of this chapter, you'll feel comfortable with the idea of using the plants that grow around you to heal yourself and your family. If you live in an urban setting and cannot harvest plants in a nearby wild space or grow your own, you can purchase plants through reputable suppliers (see the Resources section on page 227 for a list of recommendations).

Natural Health with Herbalism

Have you ever wondered how cherry became the chosen cough syrup flavor? Where aspirin got its name? Or why ginger ale is such a popular soda for upset stomachs? It might surprise you that these three products were all created from herbs.

Wild cherry bark is a great cough suppressant. Aspirin was originally made from meadowsweet (*Spiraea alba*), and ginger was traditionally used to soothe nausea and upset stomachs. Long before pharmaceutical medications, people from all cultures and walks of life relied on the healing power of herbs to remedy common ailments.

From Traditional Chinese Medicine and Indian Ayurveda to Native American healing practices, herbal medicine was the *only* medicine for centuries in cultures across the globe. In fact, according to journalist and herbalism researcher Barbara Griggs, there is evidence dating back 60,000 years in Iraq of the cultivation and application of seven species of flowering plants that are still used for medicinal purposes today.

Recipes using herbs for medicinal purposes have been passed down through countless generations of families and communities throughout the world. And even when early medical advances pushed plants to the sidelines, famous herbalism practitioners—including mystic and writer Hildegard of Bingen in the late eleventh century, physician and alchemist Paracelsus (1493–1541), and barber-surgeon John Gerard (1545–1612)—continued to write about their experiences using herbs as medicine.

Now, though the number of prescription medicines has increased dramatically in the past 40 years, the quality of healing in general has started to decline. Side effects and interactions among medications and with foods have started to leave people frustrated, in poor health, and with a quality of life that revolves around their medication schedules. There has to be a better way, right? Yes!

While medications are often given to mask symptoms, herbs used in conjunction with dietary and lifestyle changes address the cause of illness and enable people to heal and live healthy, happy lives. People are rediscovering how good it feels to bring herbs into their everyday activities for positive, long-lasting change. Herbs can be strong and effective while also being gentle enough even for children, pregnant and nursing moms, and individuals with compromised immune systems.

But herbs aren't only for those who are already ailing. They can help regain balance in the body, prevent disease, maximize health, and heal acute conditions such as bee stings, cuts, scrapes, and sprains.

If you have any fears about herbs and their potential side effects, I am here to reassure you that herbs are safe when used wisely. You may not know this, but the majority of pharmaceuticals are derived from plants. While plants have a range of constituents that work together to offer gentle healing, pharmaceuticals generally concentrate on just one plant constituent, often creating a harsher product with a whole range of side effects. Of course, there are herbs that are potent and even dangerous if taken in the wrong dose, but the herbs in this book are gentle and cause very few side effects, if any, when used correctly.

Having said that, it's important to start with the lowest dose the first time you use any herb. If you tend to be sensitive to foods and medications, start with half or even one-quarter of the suggested dose, then work your way up over the course of a few days or a week. Always read the recommended doses listed for each herb and remedy, and do not take more than suggested.

Benefits of at-Home Herbalism

There are many benefits to using herbal medicine for you and your family's health needs. For example, willow contains salicin, an anti-inflammatory that turns to salicylic acid, the primary ingredient in aspirin, when digested. Long-term use of aspirin can cause stomach ulcers, but when you use willow instead, this herb's other constituents help buffer the salicin and can actually help heal stomach ulcers.

Just like the plants we eat for nutrition, herbs also contain vitamins and minerals. For instance, dandelion flowers and roots, which are used to treat a wide variety of ailments, from skin irritations to intestinal issues, are rich in immune-boosting antioxidants and soluble fiber, respectively, and their leaves contain high amounts of vitamins A, C, and K. When incorporating herbs into our lives, we can include them in our food to provide nourishment *and* medicine.

Medicinal herbs are generally a lot less expensive than conventional medications. A bottle of cough syrup full of artificial colors and flavors may cost up to $10 (sometimes more) at your local drug store, but for a fraction of the cost, you can make an effective—and much healthier—homemade cough syrup using simple herbal ingredients from your backyard and kitchen.

❧ CONVENTIONAL VS. HERBAL MEDICINE ❧

Herbal medicine does not replace conventional medicine; they each have a place in the world of healing, and we are fortunate to have medical help in times of crisis.

While I might use herbs to help heal a broken bone, I would first want to seek the assistance of a qualified health practitioner to ensure that the bone has been set properly. And if a loved one suffered a heart attack, I would get them to a hospital immediately before turning to herbs to help rebuild and strengthen the heart against future attacks.

Some conditions, such as type 1 diabetes, cannot be healed with herbal medicine, though herbs can help support the body along with conventional treatment.

Anyone with a life-threatening illness needs the guidance of a qualified health care practitioner before incorporating herbalism into their treatment plan. Before starting an herbal regimen, it is also important to understand your condition, including its causes and symptoms, so you will be able to recognize any changes to your condition and can determine if you need medical assistance.

Herbal medicine is great for everyday bumps and scrapes and many other health conditions, as long as it is used judiciously. Though this book is a great starting point, if you have a more serious illness, consider contacting an herbalist to design a protocol specifically for you. Always seek the advice of a health care practitioner before starting an herbal treatment if you are on prescription medications and/or if symptoms seem to worsen or persist for more than 5 days after herbal treatment.

Herbs and pharmaceuticals can work together, but it is important to consult with professionals—a qualified health practitioner and herbalist—when you are taking both at the same time. Herbalists often work together with doctors, chiropractors, naturopaths, and dentists to create protocols that suit individual needs.

The initial cost of herbs may seem a bit steep. However, once you've stocked your pantry with homemade syrups, tinctures, salves, and teas, you'll see a big return on your investment over the course of a year or much longer. Don't get discouraged if you can't afford to buy every herb mentioned in this book before you start your herbalism journey. Chances are great that you don't need them all. Just pick a few recipes that correspond with the top two or three common health issues in your household, and buy the herbs for those recipes. Over time, you can continue to build your herbal pantry.

Medicinal herbs, which range from low-dose to high-dose treatments, also tend to have fewer side effects than pharmaceuticals. Low-dose herbal remedies are typically taken in small drops (1 to 10 drops at a time); high-dose herbal remedies are taken in larger amounts (40 to 60 drops at a time). You'll see both types of herbal remedies in this book, from poke (a low-dose botanical) to stinging nettles (a high-dose botanical).

Herbs in the high-dose range can generally be taken long term in large amounts without any side effects. Herbs in the low-dose range are usually more potent. Large amounts of low-dose botanicals may cause some miserable side effects, such as dizziness or vomiting. If that happens, simply stop taking the remedy and the side effects should quickly subside.

I understand any hesitation you may have about taking large doses of herbal remedies. If you're like me, you don't want to feel worse when you are trying to feel better. As long as you do your research and follow the guidelines in this book, all will be well. Take a moment to read about the herbs before using them, and seek out reliable resources for information. (See the Resources section on page 227 for more information.)

By following the recipes in this book, you'll discover cost-effective relief for a wide range of common ailments—from cuts, bruises, and insect bites to indigestion, allergies, and ringworm. You'll also learn how easy it is to incorporate healing plants into your daily routine.

How Do You Take Herbal Medicine?

Herbs work with our bodies on many levels. Just like fruits and vegetables provide us with vitamins, minerals, and other nutrients to keep us strong and healthy, herbs support us, too, with a variety of whole and natural constituents. They strengthen the immune system and are easier on our bodies than chemical-based pharmaceuticals. Just as important, viruses and bacteria don't develop immunity to herbal medicine, as they do to antibiotics.

There are a variety of ways to take herbal medicine. Here are a few of the most common types of botanical remedies:

Alcohol and vinegar-based remedies: One of the most familiar forms of herbal medicine are alcohol-based tinctures (herbs steeped in alcohol to draw out the medicinal properties), which are easy to make at home and can also be found in health food stores and online. Tinctures are simple to take because they come in bottles with droppers that allow you to add a specific amount to a cup of water or juice. Herb-infused vinegars are made in similar ways to alcohol-based tinctures and are especially useful for treating ailments such as athlete's foot fungus.

Water-based remedies: Teas and water-based decoctions and infusions are some of the easiest to make at home, whether you simply add boiling water to herbs or simmer the herbs in water. Teas can be frozen into Popsicles for children or used to create herbal baths.

Syrups: Even cough syrups are easy to make at home, and they are a great way to turn herbs into a tasty remedy for children. As Mary Poppins sang, "Just a spoonful of sugar helps the medicine go down!"

Powders: In Traditional Chinese Medicine, herbs often are ground into powders and used to make teas or pressed into tablets. Herbalists around the world use herb powders topically to staunch bleeding, seal wounds, and dry up weepy sores, among other applications.

Poultices, compresses, and massage oils: Herbs also may be applied directly to the body as poultices and compresses to aid skin conditions, sprains and strains, and fractures, and to help draw out splinters. Herb-infused oils are great for massaging herbs into the body to heal injuries such as sprains, and beeswax-based herbal salves help relieve bruises, bumps, and cuts closer to the skin's surface.

As you can see, there are lots of ways for you to use herbal medicine! But first, let's make sure you have all the supplies you need.

CHAPTER TWO

THE STARTER PANTRY

Starting any new hobby, diet, or even exercise routine can often mean spending a lot of money on the prerequisites. The great thing about learning how to heal with plants, especially herbs that grow nearby, is that you can often begin without having to make a lot of purchases. In this chapter, you'll discover how easy and affordable it is to build a powerful herbal pantry.

Most herbs in this book are easy to find or grow yourself. If you don't have a yard, many of the herbs can be grown in containers on a patio or in a sunny window. Many more can be found locally in parks, conservation sites, and other overgrown areas.

If you don't have access to green spaces where herbs may grow, there are some great companies that offer high-quality, organic, and sustainably harvested herbs at reasonable prices. (See the Resources section on page 227 for some good foraging books and my recommended suppliers.) If you have to buy your herbs in bulk, the initial investment will be more than worth it, since you'll be able to use the herbs for a year or longer depending on the kinds of remedies you make.

The tools you'll need to make herbal remedies are most likely already in your kitchen or pantry, and miscellaneous ingredients can be found at your local grocery store. Don't feel like you have to splurge on everything right away. Take your time, and discover what you most enjoy!

Getting Started

Tea is the easiest and cheapest first foray into herbalism—all you need are herbs and water! Once you've mastered teas, you may want to try making some herbal oils and vinegars. Oil- and vinegar-based treatments are another easy way to begin, since all the ingredients you need are likely already in your kitchen or pantry. These three types of remedies—herbal teas and infused vinegars and oils—can go a long way to help with everyday ailments.

When you're ready to expand your horizons, you'll want to invest in a few staples such as dropper bottles, beeswax, grain alcohol, and herbs that you can't find growing nearby. While the cost of some items (grain alcohol) can seem pricey, your tinctures will last for years.

In chapter 3, you'll learn how to make these herbal preparations and more, including decoctions (which involve simmering herbs), infusions, syrups, and salves. As you become familiar with various techniques, you'll watch your herbal pantry grow, along with your knowledge of herbal medicine.

What You'll Need

Are you ready to get started? Let's take a look at what you'll need to begin using herbs in your home and preparing the recipes in this book.

I've tried to provide enough detail so you'll know the function of each tool or ingredient. If you are not ready to create some of the more labor-intensive recipes (salves or creams), feel free to focus on making teas, vinegars, and oils. Many of the recipes offer variations and suggestions for making the process simpler. If you're not ready to make tinctures, for instance, try the same recipes as tea blends instead.

TOOLS

The following tools are listed in order of frequency of use (i.e., what you'll need the most to what you'll need the least). There are a few nice-to-have items at the end of the list, which make things easier (and replace other tools) but are not required.

Glass jars: A variety of jars from 4- to 64-ounce sizes are useful, though 8- to 12-ounce jars will be the most commonly used for preparing base tinctures, oils, and vinegars. Save empty glass food jars, or purchase canning jars for making and storing tinctures, oils, vinegars, and syrups. Be sure the lids seal tight—you don't want any leaks!

Dropper bottles: You'll need a variety of sizes from 1 to 8 ounces to dose tincture formulas. You may prefer to start with 1- or 2-ounce bottles and add larger sizes later.

Glass measuring cups and spoons: The 1-, 2-, and 4-cup sizes come in handy for measuring liquids. I prefer glass over plastic because they are clear and better for you than plastic. If you're on a budget, start with 1-cup and 4-cup sizes.

Strainer: You'll want a strainer to separate herbs from the menstruum (the liquid that is used to draw out the herb's constituents). A metal fine-mesh strainer is perfect for this job. Find several strainers in different sizes that sit comfortably over your glass measuring cups.

Labels: Always label your herbal remedies! It's important to write down what you made, when you made it, and the list of ingredients for easy identification. If you're labeling a formula or blend, you'll also want to list the instructions for how to use it. You can use sticker labels or a piece of paper with clear packing tape. (I cover my sticker labels with clear packing tape to help protect the ink from the alcohol because I often make a mess when I pour.)

Spatulas: Good for helping scrape out oils, salves, and creams. I have a regular-size silicone spatula, which I prefer, but the smaller ones are nice, too.

Ladles: These are handy for transferring liquids to containers. It helps to have a variety of sizes, from 1 tablespoon to ½ cup. The tablespoon size is a good one to start out with because it's small enough to ladle into tincture jars but still large enough for oils and salves.

Spoons: For stirring ingredients.

Thin cloth: Some people prefer cheesecloth, but I prefer Gerber pre-fold diapers. They are thin, durable, and come in large rectangles that can be cut down to the size you need. Alternatively, old T-shirts that are thin and clean can be used for lining strainers and compresses.

Cutting board: Needed to chop fresh herbs.

Sharp knife or ulu: An ulu is an all-purpose Inuit cutting tool that is rounded with a handle. I love ulus for chopping herbs, but a sharp knife works great, too. Ulus can be purchased online.

Muslin bags, tea infusers, or a tea ball: For brewing tea. Alternatively, you can use a small fine mesh strainer.

Measuring cups and spoons: For measuring ingredients.

Double boiler or saucepan: You'll need a double boiler of some kind to infuse oils, whether it's an actual double boiler or a glass measuring cup in a saucepan. I generally use a glass measuring cup when I'm making lip balm so it's easier to pour the balm into tiny tubes.

Oven mitts: Necessary to take hot items off the stove.

Waxed paper: Place waxed paper between your jar and lid when making vinegar tinctures to keep the vinegar from eroding the metal lids.

Self-adhesive elastic bandages: These are helpful for securing herbal poultices used for wounds or injuries.

Scale: A small kitchen scale is necessary to measure ingredients that are listed by weight (such as for lip balms and salves).

Stick blender: Used for making creams.

Mortar and pestle: I have found the granite (versus glass, ceramic, or metal) mortar and pestles to be the best for grinding herbs into powders.

Spray bottles: Similar to dropper bottles, these have spray tops for applying formulas topically.

Lip balm tubes: You'll need these tubes for lip balms. They also make great travel-size salve containers. Cardboard lip balm tubes are available if you prefer not to use plastic.

Eye cups: Find these at your local drugstore for rinsing eyes with herbal teas.

NICE TO HAVE:

Glass eye cups: These can be found on eBay for a few dollars. I prefer glass to plastic because the thickness of the rim feels more comfortable.

Small metal funnels: Funnels make it super easy to fill dropper bottles.

Mini crockpot: You often can find these at thrift stores. They're handy for infusing small amounts of oil instead of having to use a double boiler on the stove top.

Neti pot: Great to have on hand if you want to try nasal infusions and rinses.

Coffee grinder: A grinder works easier than a mortar and pestle for turning herbs into powders. Be sure to dedicate one for herbs only. You don't want any coffee residue in your herbal powders.

Pasta cutter: When I ferment blackberry leaves, I love to run them first through a pasta roller and then through a pasta cutter to shred them. Alternatively, you can use a rolling pin and knife.

Latex gloves: Use when handling black walnut hulls to avoid stains.

INGREDIENTS

Besides the basic herbs and tools, many recipes will require additional ingredients, which are listed here in order from most to least commonly used. (See the Resources section on page 227 for recommendations about where to purchase some of the less common ingredients.)

Grain alcohol: Gem Clear and Everclear are two common brands. If you're unable to get grain alcohol in your state, look for 100 proof vodka or ask your local liquor store to order it if they don't have it in stock. Grain alcohol, which is 95 percent alcohol, is preferred because it can be easily diluted for herbs.

Oils: Olive, coconut, sunflower, almond, jojoba, and hemp oils are all great options to have on hand. Sunflower oil is specifically needed for Sun Care Cream (page 209), and sunflower oil and castor oil are needed for Face Cleansers (pages 210 to 212). That said, oils generally can be used interchangeably, and many people use only olive oil for all their infusions. Sunflower, almond, and jojoba oils are lighter and more easily absorbed by the skin, while hemp, coconut, and olive oils tend to be heavier and stay on skin longer.

Shea butter: Needed for Sun Care Cream (page 209) and lip balm recipes.

Beeswax: Needed to help solidify salves, lip balms, and creams.

Honey: Infused with herbs or used in elixirs, lip balms, and syrups. Try to source local honey that has not been pasteurized or otherwise heated, as the heating process kills off its beneficial enzymes.

Sugar: I prefer to use raw sugar rather than white sugar for making syrups. If you choose white sugar, look for an organic or GMO-free brand.

Vitamin E softgels: Used for helping to preserve oils.

Apple cider vinegar: Needed for making Athlete's Foot Soak (page 205) and some hair care recipes. It can be substituted for alcohol in many recipes.

Glycerin: If you prefer to make nonalcoholic tinctures, you'll need glycerin. A tiny bit is needed when tincturing reishi (page 34).

Sea salt: Useful in eye wash recipes, Bath Salts (page 202), and nasal infusions.

Activated charcoal: This ingredient can help draw out toxins; see Spider Bite (page 99) and Splinter poultices (page 100). It also helps whiten teeth when added to Tooth-Cleansing Powder (page 220).

Baking soda: Used in Natural Cream Deodorant (page 207) and Tooth-Cleansing Powder (page 220).

Arrowroot powder: Used in Chafing Powder (page 167) and Natural Cream Deodorant (page 207).

Bentonite or kaolin clay: Used in Natural Cream Deodorant (page 207).

Epsom salt: Used in Bath Salts (page 202).

Black cherry fruit concentrate: This is a concentrated extract of black cherry and is not the same as fruit juice. Health food stores and some grocery stores carry this concentrate, which is used in Iron-Building Tonic Syrup (page 154).

Blackstrap molasses: This also is used in Iron-Building Tonic Syrup (page 154).

Brandy: Add brandy to help preserve Iron-Building Tonic Syrup (page 154).

Tahini: Tahini (sesame seed butter) is used in Energy Balls (page 182). Almond butter and sunflower seed butter make especially great substitutes, but any nut or seed butter will do.

You'll want a space where you can work without worrying about spilling ingredients. Most recipes only require a foot or two of counter space and your stove top. I like to play some calm music in the background to help set the mood.

It's best to assemble your tools and ingredients before you start so you'll have everything you need on hand. There's nothing worse than discovering that you are missing a key ingredient or tool after you've already started a recipe.

Some of the recipes require tinctures and oils that must be made in advance. Oils can be made in a day, but tinctures take 4 to 6 weeks to prepare. When you've determined the recipe you want to make, identify any tinctures or oils in the ingredient list that require advance preparation.

Once you've assembled everything, it's time to get started!

HERBS

Here it is, the best for last—herbs!

I am big on using plants that grow in my own backyard or can be grown easily in my climate. Working with plants that grow around you is a great way to practice herbal medicine. They are generally abundant, easy to grow, and affordable. If you cannot find them around you, the herbs suggested in this book can be easily sourced in specialty markets and online.

In each herb profile in this section, you will learn the plant's common and botanical names, useable parts, properties, treatment applications, preparation, and dosage(s). Safety considerations also are included. Although most of these herbs are very gentle and easy to use, some require caution (e.g., in case of pregnancy or liver conditions). I've also provided the amounts of herbs and alcohol needed to make tinctures because these instructions can vary from herb to herb.

You will note that many uses are listed for each herb. As you become more comfortable working with herbs, you'll want to reread this section to find herbs that might more specifically suit your needs.

BLACKBERRY

Rubus fruticosus, R. villosus,
R. allegheniensis, R. canadensis

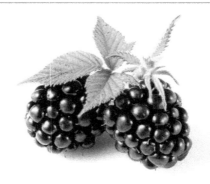

Safety considerations: Generally regarded as safe

Parts used: Leaf, root, berry

Properties: Alterative, antidiarrheal, antimicrobial, antioxidant, astringent, blood tonic, diuretic, hemostatic, muscle building tonic, nutritive, refrigerant, uterine tonic

Uses: Blackberry root is high in iron and helps counteract anemia. The root also is used to stop diarrhea and internal and external bleeding. The fermented leaf makes a great tea that helps with muscle tone. Blackberry leaf also can be used to tone the uterus, heal sore gums, and soothe sore throats. It lowers fevers, increases the flow of urine, and protects against wrinkles and UV damage. Blackberry leaf has been found to inhibit *Helicobacter pylori, Staphylococcus aureus,* and *Vibrio cholera bacteria.*

Preparations: Roots can be chopped and tinctured 1:2 in 40 percent alcohol or made into a standard syrup. To ferment and dry the leaves: Crush them with a rolling pin and then shred them with a knife or pasta cutter, place them in a lidded jar, seal, and set in a warm place for a few days to ferment. Open the jar daily and stir. After 3 to 4 days, remove the lid, spread the leaves on a clean screen or sheet, and let them dry completely. Tincture fresh leaves 1:2 in 40 percent alcohol; tincture dried leaves 1:4 in 60 percent alcohol.

Dosage: For diarrhea, take 30 drops of root tincture every 20 minutes. For other issues, take 30 to 60 drops of leaf tincture 4 to 6 times daily. Drink 1 to 2 cups of fermented leaf tea daily after a workout to increase muscle tone.

Tip: Dig roots in the spring after a soaking rain. Harvest the fresh shoots and leaves at this time, too.

BLACK HAW
Viburnum prunifolium

Safety considerations: Generally regarded as safe, but people with aspirin allergies should use with caution because black haw may contain salicin. Large doses may cause excessive drowsiness.

Part used: Stem bark

Properties: Anti-inflammatory, antispasmodic, astringent, sedative, uterine tonic

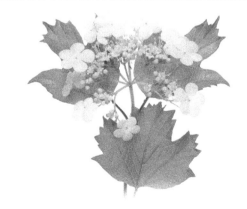

Uses: Black haw is used extensively for muscle spasms and cramping, including asthma, leg cramps, colon pain, and digestive issues. It also is used for female reproductive issues such as uterine prolapse, menstrual cramps, threatened miscarriage, nausea during pregnancy, and various types of uterine bleeding such as heavy menopausal bleeding, postnatal bleeding, and heavy bleeding during menstrual cycles.

Preparations: Tincture 1:5 in 25 percent alcohol; use dried bark for tea.

Dosage: Take 30 drops of tincture 3 times daily. For cramping, take 30 drops every 15 minutes until cramps cease. Drink 1 cup of tea as needed, up to 4 cups daily.

Tip: If you have trouble finding black haw, crampbark (*Viburnum opulus*) is a common landscape bush that can be found at many nurseries and used as an alternative.

BLACK WALNUT

Juglans nigra

Safety considerations: Generally regarded as safe

Parts used: Green and black hulls, leaves, twigs

Properties: Antibacterial, antifungal, anti-inflammatory, antiparasitic, antiseptic, antiviral, astringent, intestinal tonic, thyroid enhancer, vermifuge

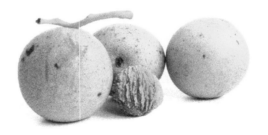

Uses: Black (rotten) hulls are used for hypothyroid conditions and goiters. Green hulls, leaf, and twig are used internally for inflammatory bowel conditions, hemorrhoids, and expelling parasites (e.g., Giardia). Black walnut is used externally for candida, ringworm and other fungi, chickenpox, and shingles outbreaks.

Preparations: Chop hulls into pieces and tincture 1:2 in 50 percent alcohol, or infuse them into a standard oil. Tincture fresh leaves and/or twigs 1:2 in 60 percent alcohol, tincture dried leaves and/or twigs 1:4 in 40 percent alcohol, or infuse them into a standard oil.

Dosage: Take 30 drops of tincture 3 times daily. Apply oil to ringworm, candida, or other infections 2 to 3 times daily.

Tip: To avoid stains, be sure to protect your hands when chopping up black walnut hulls. If you are into dyeing fabric, black walnut hulls (both green and rotten) make a beautiful dye that ranges in color from dark green to dark brown.

BURDOCK
Arctium lappa

Safety considerations: Generally regarded as safe. Use caution when separating seeds because they contain fine hairs that can irritate the skin (or lungs, if inhaled).

Parts used: Root, seeds, leaves

Properties: Adaptogen, alterative, antibacterial, antifungal, anti-inflammatory, antimicrobial (leaf), antitumor, antitussive, cholagogue, choleretic, demulcent, diaphoretic, diuretic, expectorant, febrifuge, galactagogue, hepatic, laxative, mucilaginous, nutritive, rejuvenative

Uses: Burdock leaf makes a supreme burn remedy and contains mild antimicrobial actions to prevent infection from setting into burns and wounds. Burdock root also is best for chronic conditions involving the liver. Burdock root helps restore the body to health, detoxifies the liver, increases bile production, cleanses the kidneys and bladder, and

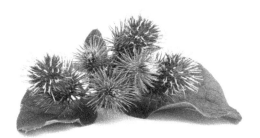

improves hormonal acne, deep cystic acne, eczema, and psoriasis, especially when used both internally and externally. The root is used in many herbal anticancer treatments, while seeds are better suited for treating acute kidney conditions, including cystitis, urinary tract inflammation, and irritated bladders. Burdock root and seed are used externally for dandruff and other scalp irritations.

Preparations: Roots can be chopped and tinctured fresh 1:2 in 60 percent alcohol or tinctured dried 1:5 in 60 percent alcohol. Dried root can be made into a standard oil or root decoction.

Seed can be crushed and tinctured 1:5 in 60 percent alcohol or used to make a standard oil infusion. Leaf can be blanched, cooled, and applied directly to burns.

Dosage: Take 30 to 90 drops of tincture 3 times daily. Drink 1 to 2 cups of decoction daily. Leaves can be applied to burns as needed, changing every 20 minutes.

Tip: Dry some leaves to have on hand during winter. Cut out the central vein, dry, then fold and roll and store in airtight jar. Burdock root is slow and deep working, so it may take up to 3 months to notice any improvement. Burdock is a biennial plant; harvest the root between the fall of the first year and the spring of the second year.

CALIFORNIA POPPY
Eschscholzia californica

Safety considerations: Do not use before driving or operating heavy equipment, as it can cause drowsiness.

Parts used: Whole flowering plant, seeds

Properties: Analgesic, anodyne, antispasmodic, anxiolytic, febrifuge, hypnotic, nervine, sedative, soporific

Uses: Used for many types of pain, especially those associated with the nervous system, including sciatica pain, nervous tension headaches, and chronic pain, when the pain can be described as hot and throbbing. California poppy calms and restores the nervous system and relieves anxiety, is gentle enough for children, and works great for overstimulated kids

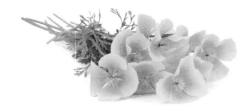

and kids with ADHD. It can help with insomnia and bedwetting associated with nervousness or tension. It's a mild febrifuge, lowering fevers, and an antispasmodic, useful for spasmodic coughs and aches associated with influenza and other respiratory conditions. The root can be placed between the gum and cheek next to a toothache for relief. Externally, the plant can be applied as a poultice or compress for relief from sciatica pain, headaches, and throbbing pain.

Preparations: Tincture fresh plant 1:1 or dried plant 1:2 in 50 percent alcohol; use dried plant for tea and compresses. Fresh root can be chewed or smashed and placed between the gum and cheek for tooth pain.

Dosage: Take 30 drops of tincture 3 times daily. For pain, take 30 drops every 30 minutes, up to 3 doses per day. Drink 1 cup of tea as needed, up to 4 cups daily. Apply compresses as needed.

Tip: Grow California poppy in containers for a lovely splash of color on your porch. If growing it in a garden, let some plants go to seed, and they will reseed for the next year.

CATNIP
Nepeta cataria

Safety considerations: Generally regarded as safe

Parts used: Aerial parts

Properties: Antidiarrheal, anti-spasmodic, antitussive, aromatic, astringent, carminative, dia-phoretic, digestive, nervine, refrigerant, sedative, mild stimulant

Uses: Catnip is gentle and effective for children and babies. As a tea, it soothes coughing spasms associated with many respiratory conditions, including bronchitis, eases cramping caused by colic and gas, and lowers fevers. Catnip is calming to the nerves and helpful for individuals who experience a fear of flying. It also reduces motion sickness and calms ADD/ADHD in children. It can be made into a spray to use as bug repellant.

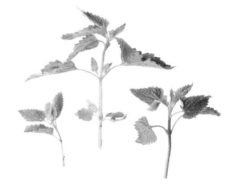

Preparations: Tincture fresh 1:2 or dried 1:5 in 50 percent alcohol, or make into standard tea.

Dosage: Take 40 to 60 drops of tincture up to 4 times daily; drink 2 to 4 cups of tea daily.

Tip: Catnip can be bitter when dried, so try adding a bit of spearmint to improve the flavor.

DANDELION

Taraxacum officinale

Safety considerations: Generally regarded as safe

Parts used: Root, leaves, flowers, stem sap

Properties: Leaves and roots are alterative, anodyne, aperient, astringent, bitter, decongestant, depurative, digestive, diuretic, galactagogue, immune stimulant, laxative, lithotriptic, nutritive, stomachic, and tonic. Additionally, leaves are antacid, antioxidant, febrifuge, hypotensive, restorative, and vulnerary. Roots also are antibacterial, antifungal, anti-inflammatory, antineoplastic, antirheumatic, cholagogue, choleretic, deobstruent, discutient, hepatic, hypnotic, purgative, and sedative. Dandelion is extremely high in many vitamins and minerals.

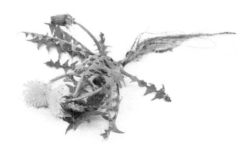

Uses: The fresh sap from the flower stem can be applied topically to remove warts and moles. The flowers are good for skin care. Dandelion is used internally in various applications for eczema, psoriasis, acne, rashes, chicken pox, shingles, measles, digestion, and constipation. It cleanses the liver; improves appetite; stimulates good bile production; stimulates the kidneys to flush fluids without depleting potassium; improves urinary issues such as urinary tract infections, bladder infections, cystitis, and kidney stones; supports stabilized blood sugar levels; and increases iron in the body. Dandelion root also has been shown to be active against leukemia, pancreatic cancer, melanoma, breast cancer, and prostate cancer.

Preparations: Tincture fresh leaves 1:1 in 75 percent alcohol; tincture dried leaves 1:4 in 50 percent alcohol. Tincture fresh root 1:2; tincture dried root 1:4 in 50 percent alcohol, or make a standard oil infusion of dried root. Infuse fresh leaf and root 1:1 in apple cider vinegar. To make leaf tea, use 1 teaspoon dried leaves per 8 ounces of boiling water and steep for 15 to 20 minutes. To make root decoction, simmer ¼ cup dried root per quart of water for 20 minutes. Dried leaf can be sprinkled on foods for added vitamin and mineral content.

Dosage: Apply fresh sap several times daily to treat warts and moles. Take 15 to 30 drops of root tincture 3 times daily, 1 tablespoon of vinegar daily, or 1 to 2 cups of tea or decoction daily.

Tip: For a deeper, coffee-like flavor, roast dried roots in a 200°F oven until they turn deep brown. Decoct or combine with cinnamon, allspice, clove, cardamom, anise, ginger, and star anise to make chai.

GINGER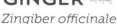
Zingiber officinale

Safety considerations: Generally regarded as safe, although it should not be taken in therapeutic doses by people who have gallbladder disease, bleed easily, and/or have a bleeding disorder or are on blood-thinning medication. It also should not be used by pregnant women with a history of miscarriage.

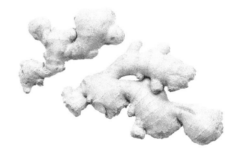

Part used: Rhizome

Properties: Analgesic, antibacterial, antiemetic, antifungal, anti-inflammatory, antioxidant, antiparasitic, antiseptic, antispasmodic, antitussive, antiviral, aperient, aphrodisiac, aromatic, cardiotonic, carminative, choleretic, circulatory stimulant, diaphoretic, emmenagogue, expectorant, febrifuge, hepatoprotective, rubefacient, sialagogue, stimulant, stomachic, vermifuge

Uses: Ginger helps to quell nausea, warming and relaxing the stomach to help with motion sickness, morning sickness, chemotherapy-induced nausea, and postoperative nausea. Ginger also helps with gas and bloating; is stimulating, bringing blood to the outer extremities and aiding poor circulation; and improves circulation in individuals with fibromyalgia to help decrease pain. Take ginger for colds and influenza to help boost the immune system, fight off viruses, soothe coughs and sore throats, expel mucus from the lungs, and sweat out a fever. Ginger is antispasmodic, relieving uterine and abdominal cramping, including cramps from irritable bowel syndrome.

Preparations: Tincture fresh rhizome 1:2 or dried 1:4 in 50 percent alcohol, or make a standard oil infusion of dried rhizome. To make a decoction, simmer ¼ cup fresh or dried rhizome per quart of water for 20 minutes. Make a standard syrup of dried or fresh root.

Dosage: Take 15 to 30 drops of tincture 3 times daily, or drink 1 to 2 cups of decoction daily. Apply oil

as needed. Take 1 to 3 teaspoons of syrup 4 to 6 times daily.

Tip: You can grow ginger in a pot in your home. Find a fresh rhizome with whitish buds at the grocery store, then set it in a sunny location until green sprouts begin to grow. Break off the section with the growth, and plant that piece in a pot. The plant will grow through spring and fall, and then it will go dormant (die back) in the winter. Set the pot in a cool (above freezing), dark location. In the spring, return it to a sunny location, water it regularly, and allow it to grow again. You should be able to harvest rhizomes in the fall.

GOLDENROD
Solidago spp.

Safety considerations: Generally regarded as safe

Parts used: Flowering tops (flowers and leaves)

Properties: Antidepressant, anti-inflammatory, aromatic, astringent, bitter, carminative, diaphoretic, diuretic, stimulant, tonic, vulnerary

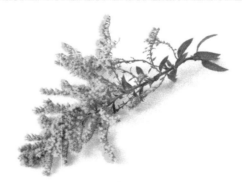

Uses: Goldenrod is helpful for pet and seasonal allergies that cause itchy, red eyes. A tea made from the flowers and leaves can stimulate digestion; relieve bloating, cramps, and gas due to sluggish digestion; soothe stomach aches and cramping accompanied by diarrhea; stimulate and tone the kidneys; reduce fevers; and lift the mood. It is especially effective for individuals suffering from seasonal affective disorder (SAD). Externally, the tea can be used to wash, disinfect, and heal wounds, and a massage oil can soothe muscle pain and strains.

Preparations: Tincture fresh flowers and/or leaves 1:2 or dried 1:5 in 50 percent alcohol, or make a standard infusion in oil. For drinking, make a standard tea. For bath tea, add 4 cups dried flower and leaf to 2 gallons water, bring to a boil, and then let steep until cool before adding to the bath.

Dosage: Take 10 to 30 drops of tincture 3 times daily, or drink 1 to 2 cups of tea daily (½ cup every hour for fevers). Massage oil into tense, strained, or painful muscles as needed.

Tip: Goldenrod often is mistaken for the flower that causes fall allergies, ragweed. For best results, harvest goldenrod when the flowers begin to open.

GOTU KOLA
Centella asiatica

Safety considerations: Generally regarded as safe, though large doses may cause dizziness, headache, itching, stupor, and vertigo. Can be stimulating to the thyroid, so avoid in cases of hyperthyroidism.

Parts used: Leaves and stems

Properties: Adaptogen, alterative, analgesic, antibacterial, anti-inflammatory, antioxidant, antirheumatic, antiseptic, antispasmodic, astringent, brain tonic, circulatory stimulant, decongestant, demulcent, depurative, diuretic, endocrine tonic, febrifuge, hypotensive, immune tonic, laxative, nervine, rejuvenative, tonic, vasodilator, vulnerary

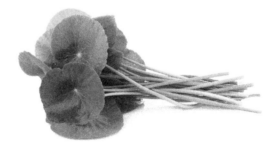

Uses: Externally, gotu kola is applied to age spots, stimulates collagen production, and heals and prevents scars, wounds, burns, bed sores, and ulcers. It also can encourage skin graft healing. Internally, gotu kola is a great brain tonic, helping to restore and improve memory and concentration, calming the mind. As a nervous system supportive, gotu kola helps with nervous breakdown, neuralgia, and depression. Gotu kola also has been used to treat ADHD, varicose veins, jaundice, macular degeneration, and other visual weaknesses. It can aid with fatigue and a wide range of diseases, including malaria, tuberculosis, syphilis, leprosy, lupus, venereal disease, and encephalitis.

Preparations: Tincture fresh leaves and stems 1:1 in 50 percent alcohol, dried 1:2 in 50 percent alcohol; use leaves and stems to make a standard infused oil. Apply dried and powdered leaves to weeping wounds and ulcers. Drink standard tea.

Dosage: Take 30 to 60 drops of tincture 3 times daily, or drink 1 to 2 cups of tea daily. Apply powder as needed.

Tip: Gotu kola is easy to grow if it has plenty of water. Plant it in a mini water garden, and keep it moist.

GROUND IVY
Glechoma hederacea

Safety considerations: Generally regarded as safe

Parts used: Aerial parts

Properties: Analgesic, anthelmintic, anti-inflammatory, antioxidant, antiseptic, antiviral, astringent, diuretic, expectorant, hepatoprotective, hypoglycemic, hypotensive, mucostatic, urinary tonic, vulnerary

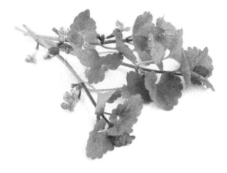

Uses: Ground ivy often is used to help flush toxic metals from the body, due to its high levels of vitamin C. It helps with tinnitus, hearing loss, otitis media with effusion or "glue ear," and ear congestion due to head colds and respiratory congestion; soothes hot, moist coughs; and eases sore throats, respiratory infections, sinusitis, and bronchitis. Ground ivy clears conjunctivitis, acute redness, itchiness, soreness, tiredness and pain in the eyes; assists with urinary issues such as gout, cystitis, urinary inflammation, urinary tract infections, kidney stones, and kidney infections; stimulates the flow of bile; and relieves intestinal cramping and diarrhea. Externally, it's applied for sciatic pain, on hot, itchy skin conditions, cuts and scratches, and on arthritis and rheumatic aches. Some studies suggest that ground ivy is beneficial for reducing plaque in the arteries, lowering blood pressure, and lowering blood glucose levels.

HAWTHORN
Crataegus spp.

Preparations: Tincture fresh 1:2 or dried 1:4 in 65 percent alcohol, or use it to make a standard tea.

Dosage: Take 15 to 30 drops of tincture up to 4 times daily, or drink 2 to 3 cups of tea daily.

Tip: Add ¼ teaspoon of sea salt to ground ivy tea, let cool, and use it as a wash to soothe tired, sore, or itchy eyes.

Safety considerations: Generally regarded as safe. Monitor blood pressure daily when taking hawthorn, as it can slow heart function.

Parts used: Berries, flowers, leaves, twigs

Properties: Adaptogen, anthelmintic, antibacterial, anti-inflammatory, antioxidant, antispasmodic, astringent, cardiotonic, carminative, circulatory stimulant, digestive, diuretic, hypotensive, lithotriptic, nervine, nutritive, rejuvenative, sedative, stimulant, trophorestorative, vasodilator

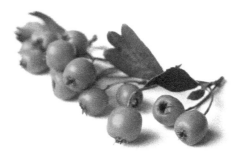

Uses: Hawthorn is terrific for all things heart-related, from grief and heartbreak to giving and receiving love. Hawthorn helps the body heal from heart attacks, heart muscle weakness, degenerative heart disease, irregular heartbeats, and congestive heart failure; stabilizes angina; and speeds recuperation from heart surgery. Hawthorn helps to open up circulation, reduces effects of hardening of the arteries, lowers blood pressure, and protects the body from free radicals that contribute to heart disease. It calms the nervous system, helps with insomnia, improves concentration and focus for children with ADD, and helps encourage speech in children with autism. It strengthens and protects joint lining, collagen, and spinal discs and also assists in the digestion of greasy food, fats, and meats. Take hawthorn immediately after getting a chiropractic adjustment to help your body hold the adjustment longer.

Preparations: Tincture berries fresh 1:2 or dried 1:5 in 60 percent alcohol; tincture flowers, leaves, and twigs fresh 1:2 or dried 1:4 in 60 percent alcohol. Make standard tea and infusion of flower, leaf, and twig.

Dosage: Take 40 to 60 drops of tincture 3 times daily, drink 1 to 3 cups of tea daily, or drink 1 to 2 cups of infusion daily.

Tip: Tincture the berry separate from the flower, leaf, and twig, but combine the two together in equal parts for a fantastic heart formula.

MILKY OATS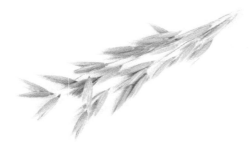
Avena sativa, A. fatua

Safety considerations: Generally regarded as safe

Parts used: Tops of oat during "milk" stage

Properties: Alterative, antidepressant, antispasmodic, demulcent, diaphoretic, diuretic, emollient, febrifuge, laxative, nervine, nutritive, rejuvenative, restorative, tonic, trophorestorative

Uses: Milky oats are high in silica and strengthening to connective tissue, skin, hair, mucosa, and nerves. As a nourishing tonic and restorative, milky oats support the endocrine, reproductive, and nervous systems, the brain, blood, and vital force in the body. Milky oat infusions help restore the nervous system; aid in healing and stress relief; ease exhaustion, insomnia, addiction to drugs (including caffeine and nicotine), and adrenal burnout; help reduce nervous palpitations, tremors, and exhaustion; and boost concentration, focus, and memory. Milky oats contain large amounts of magnesium, which helps with muscle spasms, charley horses, and other muscle cramping. A milky oat bath can be soothing for skin eruptions; hot, irritated, and itchy rashes; and conditions including poison ivy and oak, chicken pox and shingles, eczema, and sunburns.

Preparations: Tincture fresh milky oats 1:2 in 65 percent alcohol, or make a standard infusion of fresh or freshly dried tops. For an oat-meal bath, grind milky oats to a paste or powder, then transfer them to a muslin bag. Run the bag under water in the bath, then squeeze the bag to apply the "goo" to the skin.

Dosage: Take 20 to 30 drops of tincture 3 times daily, or drink 1 to 2 cups of infusion daily

Tip: If you have a sunny garden patch, try growing your own milky oats! They are easy to grow, and a 10-by-10-foot plot will yield a substantial amount. To harvest, check the tops after they flower by squeezing one of them. If a drop or two of milk comes out, they are ready to harvest. Wrap your hand around several stalks and pull up, stripping the heads from the stalks.

MONARDA
Monarda fistulosa, M. didyma, M. punctata

Safety considerations: Generally regarded as safe

Parts used: Flowering tops

Properties: Antibacterial, anti-fungal, anti-inflammatory, antimicrobial, antiseptic, anti-spasmodic, antiviral, aromatic, carminative, diaphoretic, diuretic, emmenagogue, expectorant, nervine

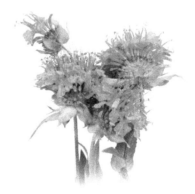

Uses: Monarda is used for diges-tive problems such as nausea, constipation, diarrhea, heart-burn, stomachaches, and gas. It is soothing for respiratory ail-ments such as colds, influenza, bronchitis, and other conditions that present with hot, spasmodic coughs. Monarda helps with chronic yeast infections that stem from leaky gut syndrome, as well as issues such as coughs, cystitis, urinary tract infections, sunburns, burns, and fevers. Monarda is one of the best herbs for reducing the symptoms of tinnitus, often with almost immediate effects. Use it as a wound wash to disinfect and encourage healing.

Preparations: Tincture fresh 1:2 or dried 1:4 in 65 percent alcohol, or use it to make a standard tea.

Dosage: For tinnitus, drop doses are most effective: 3 drops 3 times a day. For all other issues, take 30 drops of tincture 3 times a day, or drink 1 to 2 cups of tea daily.

Tip: This is a great pollinator plant with a striking flower that makes a great addition to a garden. *M. fistulosa* flowers are a beautiful pale lavender color, and the *M. didyma* flowers are show-stoppers in red or fuchsia.

MOTHERWORT
Leonurus cardiaca

Safety considerations: Generally regarded as safe, though pregnant women should avoid motherwort because of its uterine stimulant action.

Parts used: Aerial parts

Properties: Analgesic, antibacterial, antifungal, antioxidant, antirheumatic, antispasmodic, astringent, bitter, cardiotonic, circulatory stimulant, diaphoretic, diuretic, emmenagogue, hemostatic, hypotensive, immune stimulant, laxative, nervine, parturient, sedative, stomachic, tonic, uterine tonic, vasodilator

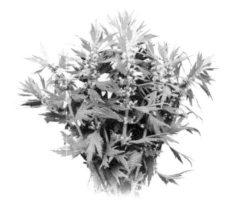

Uses: As the common name applies, motherwort is an herb for mothers; it supports the release of tension and irritation due to hormonal changes and premenstrual syndrome. Motherwort balances hormonal fluctuations for young women and elder women during the starting and ending of menstrual cycles; helps calm hot flashes, night sweats, heart palpitations, insomnia, and depression during menopause; and can reduce stress for women during childbirth. It is a uterine tonic, helpful for supporting and toning the uterus at all stages of life and even bringing on delayed menses. Motherwort softens extreme emotional upset and helps to tone the male reproductive system, too. Its botanical name, *Leonurus cardiaca*, which means "lion hearted," indicates another use of motherwort: heart health. Motherwort strengthens the heart muscle, calms palpitations, relaxes the heart, can slow a rapid heartbeat, and improves circulation. Motherwort also calms spasmodic conditions of the respiratory system, such as asthma.

Preparations: Tincture fresh 1:2 or dried 1:4 in 65 percent alcohol, or use it to make a standard tea.

Dosage: Take 10 to 30 drops of tincture 3 times a day, or drink 1 cup of tea daily (sweetened with honey, if desired).

Tip: Be careful when harvesting the flowering tops—they are quite spiny! You may wish to use gardening gloves to hold the stalks while clipping them to protect yourself from any startling pokes.

MUGWORT
Artemisia vulgaris

Safety considerations: Pregnant women should avoid mugwort, as it can cause uterine stimulation. Lactating women may find mugwort too drying. Long-term use may irritate the liver, so individuals with liver issues should avoid mugwort. If you are allergic to Asteraceae family plants, use mugwort with caution.

Parts used: Leaves, root

Properties: Analgesic, anthelmintic, antibacterial, antifungal, anti-inflammatory, antirheumatic, antiseptic, antispasmodic, antivenomous, aromatic, astringent, bitter, carminative, cholagogue, choleretic, diaphoretic, digestive,

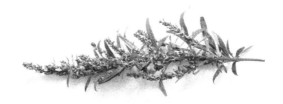

disinfectant, diuretic, emmenagogue, expectorant, hemostatic, nervine, oneirogen, purgative, stomachic, uterine stimulant, vermifuge

Uses: Mugwort eases intestinal cramping from bad digestion, food allergies and spastic colon, diarrhea, constipation, cramping, and spastic bowels. It also stimulates bile production and expels worms. In terms of reproductive health, mugwort brings on delayed menses, slows heavy menses, and relieves uterine cramping during menses. Mugwort has been shown to be helpful for individuals with dyslexia, learning disabilities, and excessive daydreams, and those who are easily distracted. Mugwort was traditionally used to help sweat out fevers and works well for intermittent fevers. As an antibacterial, mugwort is effective against a number of bacteria, including dysentery, *E. coli, Staphococcus aureus,* and strep infections. Mugwort is stimulating to the circulatory system, bringing circulation to the outer extremities for those with cold hands and feet, and it stimulates stiffness caused by rheumatism. Externally, it can be used as a wash for poison ivy and other weepy skin rashes, including eczema and psoriasis. The root has been used to reduce seizures, including those from epilepsy.

Preparations: Tincture fresh 1:2 or dried 1:5 in 50 percent alcohol, or make a vinegar extraction with fresh plant 1:1.

Dosage: Take 10 to 25 drops of tincture 3 times a day; for an acute episode, take 30 drops every 20 minutes. One tablespoon of vinegar can be taken daily, added to water or used as a salad dressing base to help with digestive issues.

Tip: For the highest potency, harvest mugwort right before it flowers. Mugwort is a dream enhancer and will make your dreams more vivid.

PLANTAIN

Plantago spp.

Safety considerations: Generally regarded as safe

Parts used: Leaves, seeds

Properties: Alterative, antibacterial, anti-inflammatory, antiseptic, anthelmintic, antivenomous, astringent, decongestant, demulcent, deobstruent, depurative, diuretic, expectorant, febrifuge, hemostatic, kidney tonic,

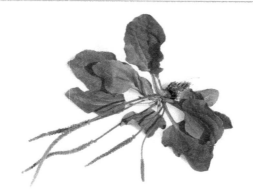

mucilaginous, ophthalmic, refrigerant, restorative, styptic, vulnerary

Uses: The seed husks (psyllium) of many *Plantago* species are used commercially for constipation. Externally, the leaves are used for insect stings and bites, typically applied as a spit poultice, as well as for cuts and nosebleeds and splinters of every kind. Internally, plantain helps stop internal bleeding and heals ulcers. For hot, dry coughs, plantain will help expectorate mucus and dry particles from the lungs and alleviate dry, ticklish coughs. Add plantain to a neti pot infusion for flushing sinus congestion, or add it to an eye wash for conjunctivitis and allergies to soothe itching, irritation and burning. Plantain tea is helpful for digestive issues (leaky gut, irritable bowel syndrome, and other intestinal problems) and urinary issues (bladder and kidney infections), and it can also be used to reduce swelling, cool heat, and heal inflammation.

Preparations: Tincture fresh leaf 1:1 in 50 percent alcohol; tincture dried leaf 1:4 in 50 percent alcohol.

Infuse freshly wilted or dried leaf in standard oil infusion. Standard tea can be made from fresh or dried leaves. For a neti pot tea, add ¼ teaspoon sea salt to hot tea and stir to dissolve. Make a spit poultice for stings, cuts, etc. by chewing fresh leaves.

Dosage: Take 15 to 30 drops of tincture 3 times daily, or drink 1 to 2 cups of tea daily or as needed for coughs and dry, ticklish lungs. Apply spit poultices to splinters, stings, cuts, and bites, repeating every 20 to 30 minutes or as needed.

Tip: If you have a splinter, chew a bit of plantain leaf, apply it to the splinter, and cover it with a Band-Aid. Change the plantain 2 to 3 times a day, and the splinter should come to the surface of the skin in a few days, depending on how long it is and how deeply it's imbedded.

PRUNELLA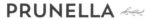
Prunella vulgaris

Safety considerations: Generally regarded as safe

Parts used: Flowering tops

Properties: Alterative, antibacterial, antibiotic, anti-inflammatory, antilithic, antimutagenic, antioxidant, antiseptic, antispasmodic, antiviral, astringent, bitter, carminative, cholagogue, diuretic, febrifuge, hemostatic, hypotensive, immune stimulant, liver stimulant, stomachic, tonic, vasodilator, vermifuge, vulnerary

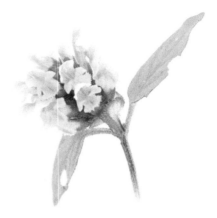

Uses: Prunella is healing for bumps, blows, bruises, cuts, sprains, strains, and scrapes. It is also an antiviral, effective in addressing colds, influenza, and other viral infections, as well as the herpes simplex virus, including cold sores and ulcers in the mouth. Prunella is an immune stimulant and fever reducer. Studies have shown that prunella has antimutagenic and antitumor properties, stopping the growth of tumors and mutagenic cells that can cause cancer. It also is useful during chemo and radiation therapy to help buffer unpleasant side effects. A tea or tincture of prunella prevents and expels gas, improves stomach function, increases the appetite, and stimulates the liver and bile flow. Prunella can help stop bleeding and prevent blood vessels from hemorrhaging. Use prunella for allergies, and apply it as an eye wash for eye issues including pinkeye and styes. Prunella also is taken to lower blood pressure, flush sodium and water from the kidneys, and restore health to the body.

Preparations: Tincture fresh tops 1:2 or dried 1:4 in 50 percent alcohol, or use dried tops to make a standard oil infusion. A standard tea can be taken internally or applied externally as an eye wash when combined with sea salt.

Dosage: Take 30 to 60 drops of tincture 3 times daily, or drink 1 to 2 cups of tea daily. Use as an eye wash as needed.

Tip: I prefer to harvest the whole tops as they are flowering, but Traditional Chinese Medicine practitioners harvest prunella when the flowering tops turn brown.

QUEEN ANNE'S LACE
Daucus carota

Safety considerations: Generally regarded as safe, but should be avoided during pregnancy, as it can cause stimulation to the uterus

Parts used: Whole plant, including flowering tops, leaf, seed (both green and brown), and root

Properties: Anthelmintic, antibacterial, anticatarrhal, anti-inflammatory, antilithic, antirheumatic, antiseptic, antispasmodic, aperient, appetite stimulant, astringent, carminative, cholagogue, contraceptive, decongestant, demulcent, diaphoretic, diuretic, emmenagogue, estrogenic, hypocholesterolemic, hypoglycemic, nervine, prostatic, relaxant, restorative, stimulant, vulnerary

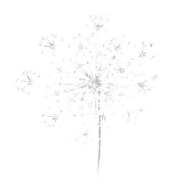

Uses: Queen Anne's lace has been used to address endometriosis and, controversially, as a contraceptive. It has been shown to help regulate the menstrual cycle, reduce heavy flows, tone the uterus while removing excessive uterine membrane growth, and dispel the placenta after childbirth. Queen Anne's lace can help balance the thyroid and pituitary glands, and is often used to reduce water retention, edema, weight gain and "beer belly," puffy eyes, fatigue related to water retention, and swollen feet. In the urinary system, Queen Anne's lace helps to remove gravel, stones, and the buildup of uric acid, and it also has been used for chronic nephritis, anuria, urinary infection, incontinence, urinary dribbling, difficult urination, smelly urine, skin rashes, cystitis, eczema, and chronic boils. Queen Anne's lace is useful for individuals who have a hard time assimilating minerals and oils, as well as for those suffering from indigestion, gas, colic, and stomach cramps.

It can help stimulate the appetite, improve bowel movements and flow of bile, and expel many types of worms, including threadworms/pinworms, roundworms, and tapeworms. It lowers blood sugar and cholesterol, expels mucus from the lungs, calms chronic coughs that are cold and wet, reduces fever, eases muscle aches and knotty muscles, and works especially well on muscles that tire easily and in individuals with fibromyalgia. Externally, Queen Anne's lace is used on tumors, sores, abscesses, carbuncles, gangrene ulcers, chronic itchy skin, dry skin, and swelling. It also promotes tissue repair, helps to granulate skin tissue to initiate healing, and kills infection in wounds.

Preparations: Tincture whole plant 1:2 or dried plant 1:5 in 60 percent alcohol, or use any part of the plant to make a standard tea or oil infusion.

Dosage: Take 20 to 60 drops of tincture 2 to 3 times daily. Apply the oil externally to skin issues, or use the tea as a wash. Drink 1 to 3 cups of tea daily.

Tip: Queen Anne's lace is the wild version of the cultivated garden carrot. It can be easily grown from seed, preferring full sun to part shade, and it will freely self-seed once established.

REISHI
Ganoderma spp.

Safety considerations: Generally regarded as safe

Parts used: Fruiting body

Properties: Adaptogen, analgesic, antibacterial, antihistamine, anti-inflammatory, antioxidant, antitumor, antitussive, antiviral, cardiotonic, expectorant, hepatoprotective, hypotensive, immune stimulant, immunomodulator, rejuvenative

Uses: As an adaptogen, reishi helps our bodies handle stress

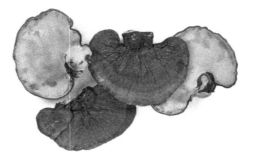

and normalize general functions. Reishi is safe to be taken long term, and it is often used to rejuvenate the body after long and/or chronic illnesses and other debilitating ailments. Reishi works to nourish and tonify, and its hepatoprotective properties help remove toxins, repair liver damage, and keep the liver healthy and strong. Reishi has been used as an antidote for mushroom poisoning and as a treatment for eczema, psoriasis, and other skin disorders through its liver-supporting action. This herb is used to help kill cancer cells, has antitumor properties, and protects against radiation exposure by protecting normal cells from radiation-related damage. Reishi controls blood sugar levels and reduces stickiness in the blood, which helps reduce the risk of stroke, lower blood pressure, and tonify and strengthen the heart. As an immune stimulant and immunomodulator, reishi is wonderful for working with immune system imbalances, including both hypo-immune conditions, such as HIV or cancer, and hyper-immune conditions, such as autoimmune diseases and allergies.

Reishi has been shown to stop serious allergic reactions, including those associated with seasonal allergies, animal dander, pollen, and chemical sensitivities, seeming to have a cumulative effect (the more you consume, the less you need). Take reishi to help promote restful sleep, relieve anxiety, enhance athletic performance, and combat altitude sickness. Reishi reduces inflammation for those suffering from arthritis, calms the respiratory system during bouts of asthma and bronchitis, helps your body fight off viruses and bacteria including *Staphylococci*, *Streptococci*, and *Bacillus pneumonia*, and has been used as a rejuvenative elixir to promote youthfulness and long life.

Preparations: Tincture fresh or dried 1:2 in a mixture of 75 percent alcohol, 20 percent glycerin, and 5 percent water in a double extraction, or use it to make a standard decoction.

Dosage: Take 40 to 60 drops of tincture 3 times daily, or drink 1 to 3 cups of decoction daily.

Tip: Replace your daily cup of coffee with a cup of reishi decoction enhanced with honey and milk.

ROSEMARY

Rosmarinus officinalis

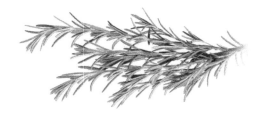

Safety considerations: Generally regarded as safe. Women with heavy menstrual flows should avoid using rosemary. Avoid during pregnancy.

Parts used: Leaves

Properties: Anodyne, antibacterial, antidepressant, antifungal, anti-inflammatory, antimicrobial, antimutagenic, antioxidant, antiseptic, antispasmodic, aromatic, astringent, bitter, cardiotonic, carminative, cephalic, cholagogue, choleretic, circulatory stimulant, diaphoretic, digestive, diuretic, emmenagogue, hypertensive, nervine, ophthalmic, rejuvenative, rubefacient, stimulant, stomachic

Uses: Rosemary stimulates the brain and circulatory and nervous systems and improves peripheral circulation and memory, making it especially useful for individuals with Alzheimer's disease. It also relieves headaches and migraines, improves vision, and may help with cataracts. As a tea, rosemary tones and calms the digestive system, improves digestion, stimulates bile production in the gall bladder and the liver, reduces fevers, relieves pain and sore muscles, brings on menstruation, and reduces high blood pressure.

Externally, rosemary is used to relieve painful sciatica pain, muscular pain, and neuralgia; decrease dandruff; darken hair when used as a hair rinse; prevent wrinkles; and ease bruising, eczema, sprains and rheumatism, and sore muscles. As a mouth freshener, rosemary cleans breath and soothes sore throats, gums, and canker sores.

Preparations: Tincture fresh 1:2 or dried 1:4 in 65 percent alcohol. A standard infusion of oil can be massaged into the body for muscle and sciatica pain or on the scalp for dandruff. A standard tea can be used to drink or as a hair rinse.

Dosage: Take 10 to 30 drops of tincture 3 to 5 times daily, or drink 1 to 2 cups of tea daily.

Tip: A good whiff of rosemary stimulates your brain function and helps wake you up. Rub it between your hands to release the essential oil.

ST. JOHN'S WORT

Hypericum perforatum

Safety considerations: Use caution when simultaneously taking prescription medications, because St. John's wort can cause the liver to process many medications more quickly. Do not take St. John's wort if you are already taking antidepressant medications.

Parts used: Flowering tops

Properties: Alterative, analgesic, anodyne, antibacterial, antibiotic, antidepressant, anti-inflammatory, antioxidant, antiseptic, antispasmodic, antiviral, anxiolytic, aromatic, astringent, cholagogue, digestive, diuretic, expectorant, nerve restorative, sedative, styptic, vermifuge, vulnerary

Uses: When applied topically, St. John's wort can work as a sunscreen and for sunburn relief. As a tincture, it relieves anxiety, depression, and seasonal affective disorder (SAD) and improves sleep quality. It can also suppress viruses such as chicken pox, herpes, and shingles. A tincture taken in the evening reduces bedwetting in children. The infused oil relieves muscle cramps such as charley horses, sciatic nerve pain, and

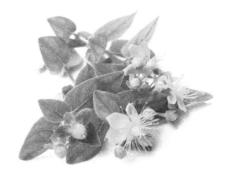

other nerve conditions. It also improves fungal issues such as *candida*, thrush, athlete's foot, and ringworm. St. John's wort may reduce nerve damage when applied topically.

Preparations: Tincture fresh flowering tops 1:2 in 65 percent alcohol or tincture freshly dried tops 1:3 in 50 percent alcohol; use fresh/freshly dried flowering tops to make a standard oil infusion.

Dosage: Take 20 to 30 drops of tincture 3 times daily. Apply the infused oil as needed 3 to 4 times daily for topical issues.

Tip: Use St. John's wort both internally and topically for best results.

SPEARMINT

Mentha spicata

Safety considerations: Generally regarded as safe

Parts used: Aerial parts of flowering plant, except stems

Properties: Analgesic, antibacterial, antiemetic, antifungal, antiviral, carminative, anti-inflammatory, antimicrobial, antiseptic, antispasmodic, aromatic, diaphoretic, nervine

Uses: Spearmint is top-notch for digestive issues, helping to calm and relax the muscles of the digestive system. Add it to tea blends to heal chronic intestinal disorders such as irritable bowel syndrome, leaky gut, and diverticulitis. Spearmint also can help relieve tension headaches, menstrual cramps, toothaches, cavities, and gingivitis. Spearmint contains menthol, which is cooling to the body. Use the tea to help lower fevers, cooling the body from the inside out. Menthol also relieves muscle spasms, coughs, and intestinal cramping. Add spearmint to a carminative tea blend to ease colic in babies.

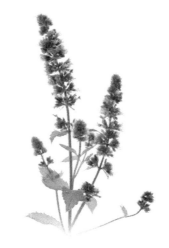

Preparations: Tincture fresh 1:2 or dried 1:4 in 65 percent alcohol. Spearmint makes a great cup of tea. Add 60 drops of tincture to 2 tablespoons water for a mouthwash.

Dosage: Take 30 to 60 drops of tincture 3 to 5 times daily, or drink 1 to 2 cups of tea as needed. Use as mouthwash 2 to 3 times daily.

Tip: Spearmint is milder and sweeter than peppermint, so it's a great herb alternative for kids.

SPILANTHES

Acmella oleracea

Safety considerations: Generally regarded as safe

Parts used: Whole plant

Properties: Analgesic, anesthetic (local), antibiotic, antifungal, anti-inflammatory, antimalarial, antimicrobial, antioxidant, antiscorbutic, antiseptic, antiviral, diuretic, febrifuge, immune stimulant, sialagogue, vasorelaxant

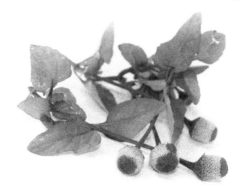

Uses: Spilanthes eases toothache pain and kills bacteria that causes periodontal disease. It also helps kill other bacteria, including *Lebsiella pneumoniae, Streptococcus mutans, E. coli, Proteus vulgaris, Pseudomonas aeruginosa, Salmonella gallinarumxi,* and *Staphylococcus albus*. Spilanthes kills other pathogens that cause herpes, tuberculosis, influenza, dengue, elephantitis, malaria, Lyme disease (best when used in the early stages), and *Candida albicans*. In addition, spilanthes improves jaundice conditions, kills worms, boosts the immune system, soothes sore throats, lowers fevers, and increases the flow of saliva.

Preparations: Tincture fresh 1:2 in 100 percent alcohol or freshly dried 1:5 in 75 percent alcohol.

Dosage: Take 30 to 60 drops of tincture 3 to 5 times daily.

Tip: I find this plant sold in my local nursery as "Eyeball Plant." Spilanthes is easy to grow from seed and does well in a container.

STINGING NETTLES 🌿

Urtica dioica

Safety considerations: Generally regarded as safe. Nettles have stingers, so harvest with caution. Avoid harvesting the leaves once the plant starts to flower; at that stage, the buildup of formic acid in the leaves may irritate the kidneys.

Parts used: Leaves, root, seeds

Properties:

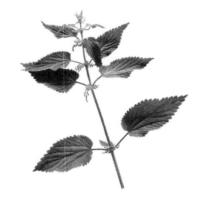

Leaves: Adrenal tonic, alterative, antiallergenic, anticatarrhal, antihistamine, anti-inflammatory, antilithic, antioxidant, antirheumatic, antiscorbutic, antiseptic, astringent, blood tonic, carminative, cholagogue, circulatory stimulant, decongestant, depurative, diuretic, expectorant, febrifuge, galactagogue, hemostatic, hypoglycemic, kidney tonic, lithotriptic, mucolytic, nervine, nutritive, parturient, pectoral, styptic, tonic, and uterine tonic.

Seeds: Adaptogen, anthelmintic, antiseptic, endocrine tonic, rejuvenative, thyroid tonic, trophorestorative, and vermifuge.

Root: Prostatic and tonic

Uses: Nettles are useful for flushing the kidneys and bladder, dissolving urinary and gall bladder stones and gravel, cleansing the kidneys and liver, and increasing kidney function. The seeds are used to energize the body and assist with kidney issues. The root is used for the prostate to help inhibit the breakdown of testosterone and can be helpful for benign prostatic hyperplasia, prostatitis, and other prostate issues. Nettle leaf nourishes the body, desensitizes against allergens, helps the liver break down allergen proteins, increases the flow of milk in nursing mothers, restores lung tissue, and contains iron and chlorophyll, which help with anemia. The stingers have been used to reduce arthritic pain and to increase circulation through direct contact.

Preparations: Tincture parts separately—fresh leaf or root 1:2 in 75 percent alcohol; dried plant or seed 1:5 in 50 percent alcohol. Use leaves to make standard infusion.

Dosage: Take 30 to 60 drops of tincture 3 to 4 times daily. Drink 1 to 2 cups of infusion daily.

THYME
Thymus vulgaris

Safety considerations: Generally regarded as safe

Parts used: Flowering tops

Properties: Anthelmintic, antibacterial, antibiotic, antifungal, antimicrobial, antiseptic, antispasmodic, antitussive, aromatic, astringent, bronchodilator, carminative, decongestant, diaphoretic, diuretic, emmenagogue, expectorant, immune tonic, rejuvenative, rubefacient, sedative (in small doses), stimulant (in large doses), vermifuge, vulnerary

Uses: Thyme works well for all respiratory conditions, both viral and bacterial. Use it for pertussis, bronchitis, colds, influenza, and pneumonia, especially with wet and spasmodic coughs. Thyme soothes sore throats and helps clear up mucus and congestion from sinusitis. Its carminative action helps babies with colic and individuals suffering from gas

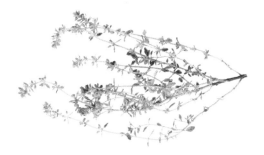

and bloating. Teas or tinctures of thyme can help expel worms like flukes and tapeworms from animal and human bodies.

Preparations: Tincture fresh 1:2 or dried 1:4 in 65 percent alcohol, or use it to make a standard tea.

Dosage: Take 30 drops of tincture 3 times a day, or drink 1 to 2 cups of tea daily.

Tip: When harvesting nettles, wear thick gloves to avoid stings. Nettle leaf is extremely nutritious and can be eaten like spinach. Nettles have hairs containing acid, but once the plant is cooked, crushed, or dried, they no longer sting.

Tip: If you suspect your child has worms, a thyme tea or tincture can help expel them. You also can add thyme to your meals to help with worm expulsion.

VITEX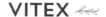
Vitex agnus-castus

Safety considerations: Generally regarded as safe

Parts used: Berries

Properties: Antispasmodic, aromatic, (mildly) astringent, diaphoretic, diuretic, emmenagogue, expectorant, febrifuge, galactagogue, ophthalmic, restorative, sedative, stomachic, vulnerary

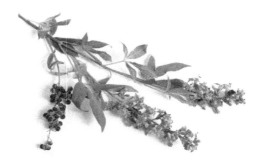

Uses: Vitex is used by both men and women to address hormonal issues, including teenage mood swings; swollen prostates; irregular menstrual cycles; breast inflammation, pain, and tenderness; and menopausal issues such as depression, lack of interest in intimacy, hot flashes and night sweats; amenorrhea, dysmenorrhea, menorrhagia, premenstrual syndrome, infertility, uterine fibroids, and ovarian cysts. In women discontinuing hormonal birth control, vitex helps rebalance hormones. Vitex also is useful for acne, including cystic acne, and many digestive issues such as gastroenteritis, indigestion, and gas. It also aids irregular bowel movements, including alternating loose stools and constipation and epigastric or abdominal pains. It helps relieve edema, spasmodic coughs, and mucus in the lungs. Vitex also can ease painful joints and muscles and help clear vision.

Preparations: Tincture 1:5 in 65 percent alcohol.

Dosage: For best results, take 60 drops of tincture in the morning, then 30 drops in the early afternoon daily. Can be added to formulas 30 to 60 drops 3 times a day.

Tip: Vitex can be slow to create changes in the body. Take it regularly for at least 3 months to see results.

WILD CHERRY

Prunus serotina

Safety considerations: May cause drowsiness. Wild cherry contains amygdalin and prunasin, which are broken down into hyrocyanic acid in the body and can be toxic in large doses.

Parts used: Bark, twigs

Properties: Antispasmodic, antitussive, astringent, bitter, carminative, diuretic, expectorant, sedative, tonic

Uses: Wild cherry is used to treat deep coughs associated with respiratory conditions such as bronchitis, pertussis, and measles. It's also great for the digestive system, often used to relieve gas and indigestion. Wild cherry can help stop panic attacks, relieve depression, and reduce the anxiety that can cause irritation, heart palpitations, restlessness, and tension headaches.

Preparations: Tincture bark 1:5 in 60 percent alcohol. Use the bark or twigs to make a standard syrup or tea.

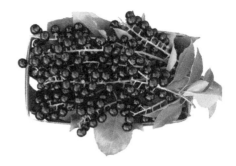

Dosage: Take 30 to 90 drops of tincture up to 4 times daily. Take 1 teaspoon of syrup as needed to treat coughs. Drink 1 to 2 cups of tea daily to ease anxiety and tension.

Tip: Turn wild cherry syrup into cough drops by heating and simmering the syrup until the liquid is reduced by half. Line a cookie sheet with waxed paper, and pour the mixture onto the waxed paper. When it cools and hardens, break it into nickel-size pieces, roll the pieces in powdered sugar, and store them in a jar.

WILD LETTUCE

Lactuca virosa

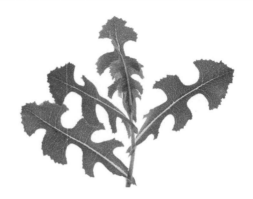

Safety considerations: Wild lettuce can be toxic if it is consumed continuously over long periods of time. Stop using it for one full week after every 4 weeks of use.

Parts used: Aerial parts, sap

Properties: Analgesic, anaphrodisiac, anodyne, antispasmodic, antitussive, digestive, diuretic, euphoriant, expectorant, febrifuge, galactagogue, hypnotic, hypoglycemic, laxative, narcotic, sedative

Uses: Wild lettuce can be used as a pain reliever for sore muscles, lower back pain, menstrual cramps, spastic colon, rheumatic pain, and other muscular pain. Wild lettuce has relaxant properties that ease cold, dry spasmodic coughs associated with respiratory complaints such as bronchitis, asthma, and pertussis. Wild lettuce helps reduce cystic acne scars and outbreaks when used over a long period of time. Some reports show that it decreases female fertility, while others suggest that it actually increases fertility, particularly among women with endometriosis. This herb increases the flow of milk in lactating mothers, calms overexcited minds, and eases pain, insomnia, and anxiety. Wild lettuce stimulates urine flow, removes edema, stimulates digestion, and relieves constipation and intestinal spasms. Externally, the sap can be used to help shrink and eliminate moles, warts, and skin tags.

Preparations: Tincture fresh aerial parts 1:2 in 95 percent alcohol.

Dosage: Take 30 to 60 drops of tincture 3 times daily. Apply sap directly to moles, warts, and skin tags several times daily.

Tip: Wild lettuce's sap seems to be the most potent right at the beginning of flowering, so harvest the tops when the first flowers bloom.

YARROW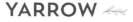
Achillea millefolium

Safety considerations: Yarrow should be not by used by anyone with a blood clotting disorder.

Parts used: Whole flowering plant

Properties: Analgesic, anodyne, antifungal, anti-inflammatory, antiseptic, antispasmodic, aromatic, astringent, carminative, cholagogue, circulatory stimulant, diaphoretic, digestive, diuretic, emmenagogue, expectorant, febrifuge, hemostatic, hypotensive, nerve relaxant, odontalgic, parturient, stimulant, stomachic, styptic, sudorific, tonic, urinary antiseptic, uterine decongestant, uterine stimulant, vasodilator, vulnerary

Uses: Yarrow can be applied topically to treat bleeding, scratches, cuts, wounds, hemorrhoids, varicose veins, oily skin, and acne. Yarrow is also consumed as a tea or used as a tincture to address internal issues, including cystitis, fevers, sluggish liver, digestive issues, fevers, and high blood pressure.

Preparations: Tincture fresh 1:2 or dried 1:5 in 50 percent alcohol. Use dried yarrow to make a standard oil infusion. Use fresh or dried

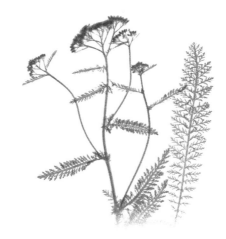

flowers to make a standard tea. Dried, powdered yarrow can be used topically to treat bleeding, weepy wounds.

Dosage: Take 10 to 40 drops of tincture internally 3 times daily. Drink 1 cup of tea as needed for fevers and urinary issues. Apply tincture externally several times daily as needed to treat acne, oily skin, and varicose veins. Apply dried, powdered yarrow directly to wounds to stop bleeding and weeping.

Tip: Try adding a pinch of spearmint or other sweet tasting herbs to help sweeten the tea's flavor.

10 BONUS HERB PROFILES

The following herbs appear in the recipes in this book, but relatively infrequently. Think of this as the "nice-to-have" list: Once your herb pantry is stocked with the most commonly used herbs, consider purchasing a few of these to round out your inventory.

BORAGE

Borago officinalis

Safety considerations: Do not use long term or if you have liver issues. Borage should not be used by pregnant women.

Parts used: Aerial parts

Properties: Adrenal tonic, alterative, anti-inflammatory, demulcent, diaphoretic, diuretic, emollient, refrigerant

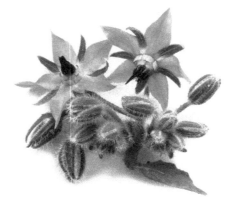

Uses: Borage has properties that can help you find courage to break through grief, depression, and worry to heal and feel better. It has been shown to reduce suffering from post-traumatic stress disorder and severe nervous exhaustion, reduce varicose veins and heart palpitations caused by hyperthyroidism, and help lower fevers and cool hot flashes and gut issues. Borage can be used externally to treat sore, puffy eyes and skin conditions.

Preparations: Tincture fresh leaf and flower 1:2 in 75 percent alcohol. Use fresh or dried leaf and/or flower to make a standard tea or compress.

Dosage: Take 10 to 30 drops of tincture 3 times daily.

CALENDULA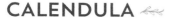
Calendula officinalis

Safety considerations: Generally regarded as safe

Parts used: Flowers

Properties: Alterative, antibacterial, antifungal, anti-inflammatory, antimicrobial, antispasmodic, antiviral, astringent, cholagogue, demulcent, diaphoretic, immune stimulant, lymphatic, vulnerary

Uses: Calendula has been shown to relieve skin conditions such as varicose veins, bleeding wounds, sores, cuts, scrapes, sunburns, insect bites, measles, and chickenpox. Calendula inhibits the growth of bacteria, stimulates liver function and bile flow, and combines well with black walnut to rid the body of fungi such as candida, thrush, and athlete's foot.

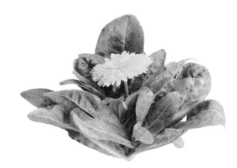

Calendula also assists in digestive healing.

Preparations: Tincture fresh flowers 1:2 or dried 1:4 in 70 percent alcohol, or use fresh or dried flowers to make a standard tea or infused oil. Use tea as a compress, or use mashed fresh flowers as a poultice.

Dosage: Take 5 to 30 drops of tincture up to 4 times daily, or drink 1 to 3 cups of tea daily.

CLEAVERS
Galium aparine

Safety considerations: Generally regarded as safe

Parts used: Aerial parts

Properties: Alterative, anti-inflammatory, antineoplastic, aperient, astringent, detoxifier, diaphoretic, diuretic, febrifuge,

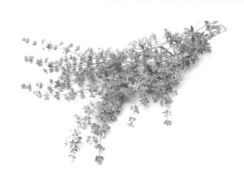

hypotensive, immune tonic, lithotriptic, lymphatic, vulnerary

Uses: This plant is especially effective in addressing lymph-related illnesses, including tonsillitis, earaches, adenoid problems, nodular growths, chronic and acute swollen lymph nodes, and breast cysts. It also helps to shrink fibroid tumors and benign or cancerous tumors; reduces outbreaks of eczema, psoriasis, and other skin issues; helps eliminate cystitis, urethritis, irritable bladder, prostatitis, urinary tract infections, and kidney inflammation; soothes nerves; and can be applied externally to scar tissue, insect bites, and slow-to-heal wounds.

Preparations: Tincture fresh leaves and stems 1:2 in 60 percent alcohol, or use the leaves and stems to make standard tea. Use the tea as a compress, or use the mashed fresh plant as a poultice.

Dosage: Take 40 to 60 drops of tincture up to 4 times a day, or drink 2 to 4 cups of tea daily.

COMFREY
Symphytum officinale

Safety considerations: Root should never be taken internally. Do not use if you have a history of liver conditions or regularly consume alcohol. Use comfrey leaves internally for short periods of time (2 to 4 weeks only). Do not use internally during pregnancy or lactation.

Parts used: Root, leaves

Properties: Alterative, anodyne, anti-inflammatory, antirheumatic, astringent, biogenic stimulator, demulcent, emollient, hemostatic, styptic, vulnerary

Uses: When applied externally, comfrey root helps reduce or eliminate scars and fade age spots. The

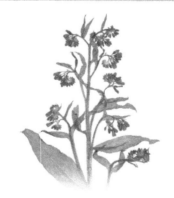

leaves can be used externally to soothe dry, itchy skin and help heal cuts, perineal tears from childbirth, broken bones, external ulcers, and wounds (when applied in combination with an antimicrobial herb to avoid infection being sealed into the wound). Comfrey leaves have been used internally to heal gastric and duodenal ulcers, ulcerative colitis, and leaky gut.

Preparations: Apply a root poultice directly to scar tissue to reduce scarring. Make a tea with ¼ cup leaves for every 8 ounces of boiling water, steeped for 20 minutes, to drink or use as a compress.

Dosage: Apply root poultices and leaf compresses 3 to 6 times daily for no longer than 6 weeks. Drink 1 cup of tea daily for no longer than 4 weeks.

LEMON BALM ✿
Melissa officinalis

Safety considerations: Generally regarded as safe. Women with a history of miscarriages should avoid therapeutic doses during pregnancy.

Parts used: Flowering tops

Properties: Antibacterial, antidepressant, anti-inflammatory, antispasmodic, antiviral, aromatic, carminative, cholagogue, diaphoretic, febrifuge, hypotensive (mild), nervine, rejuvenative, sedative, stomachic

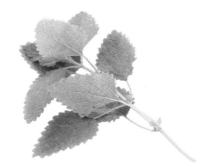

Uses: Lemon balm is commonly used for nervous system complaints, such as nervousness, anxiety, stress, headaches caused by nervous tension, and illnesses that affect the nervous system, including chronic fatigue and depression. Improves concentration and cognitive function and decreases agitation (especially for those with Alzheimer's disease, dementia, and ADHD), helps to ease stress-related digestive complaints, increases flow of bile in the liver, aids in fighting off viruses, and lowers blood pressure. When used externally, lemon balm repels mosquitoes and other insects.

Preparations: Tincture fresh tops 1:2 in 100 percent alcohol or dried 1:5 in 75 percent alcohol, or use the tops to make a standard oil infusion. For drinking, make a standard tea.

Dosage: Take 30 to 60 drops of tincture 3 times daily, or drink 3 to 4 cups of tea daily.

NEW ENGLAND ASTER ✍

Symphyotrichum novae-angliae

Safety considerations: Generally regarded as safe

Parts used: Flowers

Properties: Antispasmodic, aromatic, bronchodilator, calmative, decongestant, diaphoretic, expectorant, nervine, relaxant, stimulant

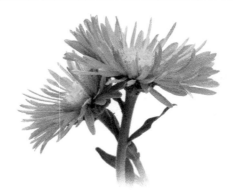

Uses: Aster can be used to help shortness of breath, congestion, asthma, allergies, colds, influenza, bronchitis, pneumonia, congestion, and coughs. It also helps calm tension and stop panic attacks, and when used preventatively, it can help lessen the intensity of asthma attacks.

Preparations: Tincture fresh flowers 1:1 in 75 percent alcohol

or dried flowers 1:2 in 60 percent alcohol.

Dosage: Take 15 to 20 drops of tincture every 20 minutes for acute situations; take 20 to 30 drops of tincture 3 times daily for preventative use.

PASSIONFLOWER ✍

Passiflora spp.

Safety considerations: Large doses may cause dizziness, nausea, and vomiting. Individuals who are pregnant, on MAO-inhibiting antidepressant medications, or have kidney disease should consult with a health care practitioner prior to use. Not recommended for children under 4.

Parts used: Aerial parts

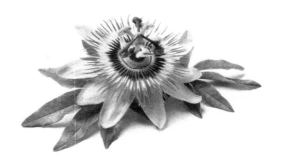

Properties: Analgesic, anodyne, antibacterial, antidepressant, antifungal, anti-inflammatory, antispasmodic, cerebral vasore-laxant, hypnotic, hypotensive, nervine, sedative

Uses: Passionflower is commonly used for depression, hysteria, pertussis, anger, stress-induced headaches, muscle tension, neuralgia, shingles, Parkinson's disease, anxiety, insomnia, ADHD/ADD, and spasms related to most bronchial ailments. It also stops hiccups, calms and eases many nervous system complaints, and can also help reduce the risk of addiction to opiate and/or benzo-diazepine medications.

Preparations: Tincture fresh plant 1:2 in 50 percent alcohol or dried 1:5 in 50 percent alcohol. Use the plant to make a standard tea.

Dosage: Take 30 to 60 drops of tincture up to 4 times daily (or every 20 minutes for an acute epi-sode), or drink 1 to 2 cups tea daily.

POKE
Phytolacca americana

Safety considerations: *Use with caution.* Excessive doses cause hallucinations, nausea, vomiting, abdominal pain, diarrhea, diffi-culty breathing, convulsions, and tachycardia. Crushed seeds are toxic. During lactation, remove thoroughly from breast before nursing. Avoid during pregnancy. If you think you've consumed too much poke, first seek medical assistance, then eat plain yogurt to help absorb the toxins.

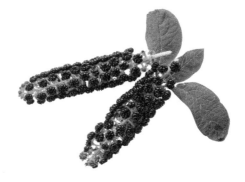

Parts used: Root, berries

Properties: Alterative, analgesic, anodyne, antibacterial, antifungal, anti-inflammatory, antirheumatic, antitumor, antiviral, cathartic, emetic, immunostimulant, lym-phatic, narcotic, purgative

Uses: The root helps drain lymph fluids and resolve mastitis. The berries, when mashed with water (a.k.a. Pink Water), help purge a lin-gering cold, causing a temporary resurgence of symptoms as they are flushed, and can be used to combat leukemia, cancer, herpes, mumps, swollen glands, tonsillitis, laryngitis, tinea, ringworm, and acne. The root can be made into a poultice or salve to be used externally for mastitis and a variety of skin issues.

Preparations: Tincture fresh root or berries 1:2 in 65 percent alcohol; tincture dried root or berries 1:5 in 50 percent alcohol. Use fresh or dried root or berries to make a standard oil infusion. To make Pink Water, add 8 berries to 1 quart water, then mash well and strain the liquid.

Dosage: Take 1 to 8 drops of tincture up to 3 times daily. Drink 2 to 4 cups of Pink Water over the course of 1 day.

SAW PALMETTO ✿
Serenoa repens

Safety considerations: Generally regarded as safe. Rarely causes stomach upset. Consult a health professional prior to use if you have prostate issues.

Parts used: Berries

Properties: Alterative, anabolic, antiandrogenic, anticatarrhal, antiestrogenic, anti-inflammatory, antiseptic, antispasmodic, decongestant, diuretic, expectorant, muscle building tonic, nutritive, phytoestrogenic, rejuvenative, reproductive amphoteric, restorative, thyroid tonic, uterine tonic

Uses: Saw palmetto can help address prostate issues, including increased urinary frequency, reduction of the urinary stream, difficulty urinating, urinary retention, and incomplete emptying of the bladder. It has also been used

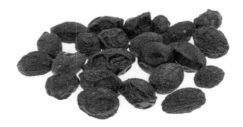

to combat male pattern baldness, polycystic ovarian disease, infertility associated with elevated estrogen and testosterone combined with low progesterone, ovarian pain, and cystic acne.

Preparations: Tincture fresh berries 1:2 or dried berries 1:5 in 80 percent alcohol.

Dosage: Take 30 to 90 drops of tincture 3 times daily.

YELLOW DOCK

Rumex crispus, R. obtusifolius

Safety considerations: Generally regarded as safe

Parts used: Root

Properties: Alterative, anti-inflammatory, antiscorbutic, antiseptic, aperient, astringent, blood tonic, cholagogue, depurative, diuretic, laxative, liver tonic, tonic

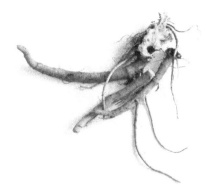

Uses: Properties in yellow dock can help the body absorb iron. This herb can also work as a laxative; aid liver function; clear jaundice, eczema, psoriasis, acne, and other skin issues; and aid in liver and gall bladder health. Yellow dock mouthwash helps kill bacteria and tone gums.

Preparations: Tincture fresh root 1:2 or dried root 1:5 in 50 percent alcohol. Use fresh or dried root to make a standard vinegar, standard decoction, or basic syrup.

Dosage: Take 30 to 80 drops of tincture 3 times daily; drink 1 to 2 cups of decoction or 3 to 6 tablespoons of infused vinegar or syrup daily to treat iron deficiency.

Where to Get Your Herbs

There are many different ways to obtain healing herbs. My favorite choice is harvesting them in the wild around my home. If you can identify plants with certainty, know that the location has not been sprayed with pesticides and/or herbicides, and have permission from the landowner, harvest away! (See the Resources section on page 227 for more information about plant identification.)

Container gardening is a great option if you don't have a backyard or community garden plot. Alternatively, seek out some of the great resources that are available online. Look for companies and individuals who grow and sell organic and sustainably grown herbs. Sustainably grown herbs are the only kind included in this book. (See the Resources section on page 227 for more information about suppliers.)

It's always best to purchase organic and sustainably grown herbs, because commercially grown and stored herbs are often sprayed with pesticides and

⇝ GROWING YOUR OWN HERBS ⇜

It's okay to buy your herbs, but if you can grow them yourself, that's even better. The quality of herbs grown at home (or harvested locally) is much higher, and the cost is low! Most of the ones listed in this book are "weedy" plants that will grow in a variety of climates without a lot of fuss.

If you have a yard, you can create a small herb patch. Chances are, too, that many herbs—including cleavers, dandelion, goldenrod, ground ivy, Queen Anne's lace, plantain, poke, prunella, wild lettuce, and yellow dock—are already present, especially if you're like me and don't spend a lot of time weeding your garden.

If you have trees around your home, you might even have hawthorn, black walnut, and wild cherry growing. If not, they are great to add to your yard.

If you live in an apartment, many plants such as spilanthes, spearmint, rosemary, St. John's wort, yarrow, calendula, and catnip can be easily grown in pots and are great for beginners. Even passionflower can be grown in a pot with a trellis. Start with just a few plants in pots, and then, as your confidence in gardening grows, so will your herb collection! (See the Resources section on page 227 for a list of seed and plant suppliers.)

herbicides. These harmful chemicals are still on the herbs when they are dried and processed and will go directly into your herbal medicine. That's not something you want to ingest when you are trying to heal!

To determine if you have purchased high-quality herbs, do a simple test. Dried herbs should be vibrant and colorful: their leaves should still be fairly green and their flowers and roots should retain their petal color (New England aster and goldenrod are exceptions, as are members of the Asteraceae family, which turn to fluff when dried). Dried herbs also should be aromatic and have a flavorful taste. Make a habit of inspecting your herbs, and keep a record of how they look, taste, and smell the day you buy them. This will help you determine later if the herb is old and ready to be composted.

Fresh vs. Dried Herbs

Fresh is not always best when it comes to using herbs. For the majority of herbs, it's best to use dried or significantly wilted fresh herbs when infusing them in oils. This is because oil and water don't mix well, and moisture from the herb in the oil will quickly turn oil rancid. Herbs such as St. John's wort and cleavers are best used fresh in oil and are exceptions to this rule.

Dried herbs are also better than fresh for making herbal honeys. That way, you don't risk adding water to your honey, which can cause it to ferment.

Some herbs, such as milky oats and wild lettuce, are always better fresh, as they lose their most beneficial constituents when they are dried.

Dried herbs are easy to store and should be kept in a sealed container away from sunlight to help them stay fresh longer. I store mine in carefully labeled glass jars in a cupboard. Typically, dried herbs will stay fresh for 1 to 2 years, depending on the specific plant.

If you are planning to dry your own fresh herbs to make tinctures, syrups, and so on, you will need to start with larger amounts of herbs than you might expect, since they shrink considerably when they are dried.

For the best color and overall vibrancy, I like to use fresh herbs to make alcohol or vinegar extractions. Stinging nettles, for example, turn an emerald green when extracted fresh.

On the other hand, dried herbs make for much more aromatic oils and infusions, as heating the dried herbs helps draw out their constituents.

❧ DRYING YOUR OWN HERBS ❧

Here are a few methods for dehydrating your own fresh herbs.

Outside: The easiest way, particularly for large amounts of herbs, is to lay them out on an old sheet in the shade (so the sun doesn't bake them to a crisp and remove their medicinal qualities).

Bunched and hung upside down: Herbs also can be gathered in bunches and hung to dry, using a rubber band to secure them at the stem ends. Hang them in a room that is fairly warm and away from direct sunlight. This method can take up to a few weeks to fully dry the herbs, and you'll want to make sure not to bundle them too thickly or they may start to mold before they dry.

Loose in baskets: Herbs also can be stashed in baskets for drying; just remember to "fluff" them daily. Gently lift herbs from the bottom of the pile to the top of the pile so that all of them circulate and dry well. Use baskets that have a bit of an open weave for herbs that are larger; use tighter-woven baskets for smaller herbs or seeds. I generally place my drying baskets on top of the fridge or bookshelves where it's warmer and out of the way of my cats and dogs.

In the oven: If your oven has a low setting, it can be used for drying herbs and works especially well for drying roots. Be sure to wash your roots well, then chop them into small pieces before drying. Some roots, such as poke, are extremely hard and impossible to chop when dried.

In a dehydrator: A dehydrator can be programmed to dry your herbs. Generally, you don't need to fluff the herbs when you dry them using this appliance, though some dehydrators work better than others.

A few notes on drying herbs: When drying large herbs such as burdock leaves, cut out the main veins so the leaves will dry evenly.

Once your herbs have dried, break them up slightly to store them in jars. I try not to crumble them or break them up too much to avoid reducing their potency. As a rule of thumb, dried leaves and flowers generally last for 1 to 2 years, while dried seeds, bark, and roots will last for up to 3 to 4 years. (Remember to label and date your herbs and remedies!) The better you store your herbs—in a dark cabinet away from sunlight and heat—the longer they will last. I always examine an herb's color, smell, and taste before I use it.

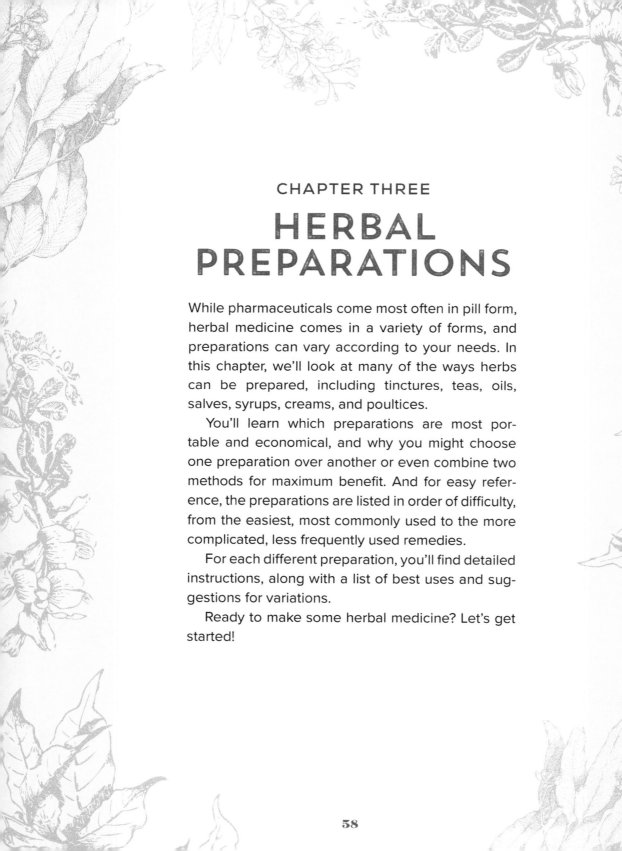

CHAPTER THREE

HERBAL PREPARATIONS

While pharmaceuticals come most often in pill form, herbal medicine comes in a variety of forms, and preparations can vary according to your needs. In this chapter, we'll look at many of the ways herbs can be prepared, including tinctures, teas, oils, salves, syrups, creams, and poultices.

You'll learn which preparations are most portable and economical, and why you might choose one preparation over another or even combine two methods for maximum benefit. And for easy reference, the preparations are listed in order of difficulty, from the easiest, most commonly used to the more complicated, less frequently used remedies.

For each different preparation, you'll find detailed instructions, along with a list of best uses and suggestions for variations.

Ready to make some herbal medicine? Let's get started!

Preparations for Different Situations

When it comes to using herbs, I like to correlate herbal medicine to the ailment as much as possible. For instance, if I've sprained my ankle, I'll use a poultice or compress directly on the sprain, possibly followed up with an oil or salve. At the same time, if I am dealing with tension and my nerves are frazzled, I find that teas and tinctures offer the most comfort.

Sometimes, however, I find it helpful to use herbs both internally and externally. For example, for an earache, I always apply Earache Oil (page 129) directly into the ear. But I also might consider boosting my immune system with the Immune System Boost & Support Tonic Elixir (page 132) to help my body fight off any lurking infection.

No recipe is set in stone. As you learn more about herbal remedies, you may want to try other herbs that might work better for you. At the same time, if a tea blend doesn't suit your tastes (or your child's), you can turn it into a tincture and follow standard dosing. Similarly, if a cream or salve recipe seems too intimidating, make the same recipe into a standard oil instead.

If you're on the go a lot, you may gravitate toward tinctures, tonics, and elixirs, which can be tucked into your purse or backpack. (Pro tip: Teas can also be made portable in a thermos or water bottle.)

For topical applications, there are many choices to choose from: poultices, compresses, oils, salves, creams, lotions, powders, and baths. Water-based preparations are less messy than oil-based preparations, though, so you'll want to take this into consideration when choosing recipes.

If you have questions about specific preparations, feel free to jump ahead to the relevant section or the glossary (see page 223) for a quick definition. Though the names for some preparations may seem odd, you'll soon understand what they are, how they are used, and how to make them, and you'll be speaking like an expert herbalist in no time!

One final thought: If you're wondering why you would want to go to the trouble of making herbal medicine when you can buy it off a store shelf, the number one reason is cost. Making your own preparations is cost-effective (you can buy a 1-ounce bottle of tincture for around $12 or make a half gallon for about the same price), and you'll be assured that the herbs are what they're supposed to be, as well as being fresh and good quality.

There are many ways to measure out your ingredients, and no one way is the only right way. Some herbalists tend to use parts (3 parts of this plus 2 parts of that), but I like to use measurements. I typically measure in volume, so you'll see all the ingredients listed in teaspoons and tablespoons, with cups for dry ingredients and ounces for liquid. The only time I use a scale is when I am measuring out ingredients for lip balms and salves, because it's hard to measure beeswax in volume.

Dosage matters, especially if you are using a low-dose botanical. When it comes to dosages, I generally refer to drops for tinctures. As you become more familiar with using tinctures, you'll notice that 30 drops often is equivalent to what is referred to as a "dropperful." I don't like to say "dropperful," because the amount varies with each herb and I want to avoid any confusion.

When determining the correct dosage, start with the lowest amount for an adult who weighs around 150 pounds, increasing or decreasing according to weight. For instance, a child who weighs 75 pounds would take half the amount of the suggested adult dosage, while a 300-pound adult would need to take double the suggested amount. This same rule applies for dosing teas. A final consideration to take into account is that an individual's health, weight, age, and sensitivity can affect how their body reacts to a remedy; lower the dosage when sensitivity is higher and/or there are health issues.

Herbal Teas

Herbal teas can be as simple as dipping a tea bag in water or as complex as simmering a combination of herbs for a specific period of time. Let's take a look at a few terms associated with tea making.

An herbal tea also can be called a *tisane* or a *diffusion*. Herbalists often use one of these names to make the distinction that a tea is herbal and not caffeinated.

A *diffusion* refers to submerging a large concentration of substance, such as dried herbs, into hot water. You may have noticed this process when you've made yourself a cup of hot black tea—the clear water turns brown as the tea diffuses into the water. A *tisane* is just another word for an herbal tea. Typically, we create a diffusion or a tisane when steeping herbal flowers, leaves, and aromatic parts in water.

To make a tisane or diffusion: *Steep 1 to 2 teaspoons of dried herb or 3 to 4 teaspoons of fresh herb in 8 to 10 ounces of hot to boiling water for 15 to 30 minutes, depending on the herbs. Most of the recipes in this book are diffusions, including the Cold Care Tea Blend (page 85) and the Anxiety Tea Blend (page 109). Strain into a mug and drink hot, or strain into a clean jar, seal, and store in the refrigerator for the next day.*

Sometimes you need to heat herbs at a consistently high temperature to draw out their medicinal properties, so you make what is known as a *decoction*. Herbs are put in a saucepan with water that is heated until it boils, and then everything is left to simmer. I typically use this method for making tea with relatively hard plant materials such as roots, barks, and seeds.

To make a decoction: *Combine 1 to 4 tablespoons of dried herbs and 12 to 16 ounces of water in a saucepan. Bring the water to a boil, then turn down the heat and simmer the mixture for 20 to 45 minutes. Strain into a mug and drink hot, or strain into a clean jar, seal, and store in the refrigerator for the next day.*

Infusions are another method of making herbal teas, and the term can mean different things to different people. I describe an infusion as a large quantity of a single herb steeped in hot water for several hours to extract its minerals. Infusions typically are used for nutritive herbs such as stinging nettles, milky oats, and hawthorn leaves and flowers.

To make an infusion: *Place 1 cup of dried herb in a quart-size jar (or 2 cups in a ½-gallon-size jar), fill the jar with boiling water, and let the mixture steep for 6 to 12 hours. Strain the liquid through a fine-mesh sieve into a clean jar; seal and refrigerate.*

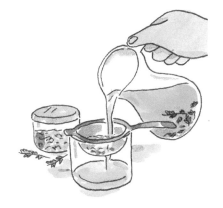

Some people like to make infusions overnight and strain them in the morning. I prefer to make mine in the morning so I can strain and chill them for the following day. Infusions will last for about 4 to 5 days in the refrigerator, and you can drink them cold, hot, or at room temperature. Infusions with bitter herbs such as hawthorn may taste better if you add a pinch of spearmint (just a pinch is all that's needed); some people find that stinging nettle infusion tastes better with an added pinch of sea salt. Try them plain first, then add other herbs as desired.

Generally, infusions are made with only one herb, whereas diffusions and decoctions can be made with multiple herbs.

Tinctures

The best-known herbal remedy is probably the *tincture*. Tinctures steep a little bit of herb in a menstruum such as alcohol or vinegar to make a lot of medicine.

An herb-infused vinegar is known as an *acetum*. Vinegar can be used in place of alcohol for tincturing some herbs, but it's not always the best solution because it doesn't always extract the medicinal properties as well as alcohol. Herbs such as dandelion, burdock, and yellow dock make great vinegar tinctures to be used on salads or consumed in water for their mineral content.

> **To make an acetum:** *Fill half a jar with chopped fresh herbs, and then top it off with vinegar. For the best results, steep the herb for 2 to 4 weeks before use, and leave the herbs in the vinegar during storage. If using dried herbs, fill the jar ¼ full with the herbs before pouring in the vinegar.*

I prefer to use apple cider vinegar because it's healthy, but any vinegar can be made into an acetum. Sometimes the vinegar is best heated up and then poured onto the herbs, such as in the recipe for Athlete's Foot Soak (page 205). This method, similar to that for making a diffusion, extracts more of the medicinal properties and less of the mineral content of the herbs.

To make alcohol *tinctures*, fresh or dried herbs are chopped, added to alcohol, and steeped for 4 to 6 weeks. Historically, red wine was used to make tinctures (as was beer, which to this day is typically made with hops, an herb that helps induce calm and sleep). But these days, we generally use grain alcohol, vodka, or brandy. I prefer to use grain alcohol so I can control the alcohol content to a greater degree, depending on the herbs I am extracting. However, brandy, because it's made from pears, which are easy on the digestive system, is nice if you are making a digestive blend.

Because alcohol content varies by herb, you'll notice in the herb profiles that instructions are provided like this: Tincture fresh 1:2 or dried 1:4 in 65 percent alcohol. Accordingly, fill any size jar with 1 part of herb (fresh) to 2 parts menstruum made up of 65 percent alcohol and 35 percent water. Alcohol and water ratios will vary by herb.

To make an alcohol tincture in an 8-ounce jar (using the 1:2 example ratio above): *Fill half your jar with chopped fresh herbs, then pour in grain alcohol until the jar is about 65 percent full and top off the jar with water. Seal the jar and let the mixture steep for 4 to 6 weeks. Strain some of the liquid through a fine-mesh sieve into a clean bottle for dosing; and discard the plant materials or return them to the jar with the rest of the tincture.*

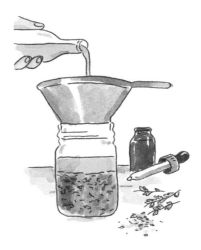

I prefer to leave hard materials such as seeds, roots, and bark in my tinctures so the medicinal properties continue to be extracted. Most tinctures will keep indefinitely, as long as they are stored in a cool, dark location.

Sometimes herbs are best tinctured in double extractions. One example of this is reishi (page 34).

To make a double-extraction tincture of reishi (see page 34):
Combine the herbs, alcohol, glycerin, and water in a jar, screw on the lid, and let the mixture steep for 4 weeks, shaking it daily. Glycerin is not always needed in a double extraction, but it is helpful for drawing out the constituents of reishi. After 4 weeks (or longer), strain the alcohol through a fine-mesh sieve into a large measuring cup or jar, and transfer the strained reishi to a saucepan.

Measure the amount of strained alcohol, and pour double that amount of water into the saucepan over the reishi. For instance, if you have 8 ounces of strained alcohol tincture, add 16 ounces of water. Bring the water to a boil, reduce the heat, and simmer the mixture for about 1 hour or until the liquid has reduced by half. Turn off the heat and allow the decoction to cool. Strain the liquid through a fine-mesh sieve into a large, clean jar, discard the reishi, and then add alcohol tincture; seal the jar and shake well to combine. Label your double extraction with all the usual information.

Be sure to shake your tinctures before every use, whether you're ingesting them directly or mixing them with other tinctures to make a blend. Tinctures will generally last indefinitely if stored in a cool, dark location. When tinctured, none of the herbs in this book lose their potency over time.

Tonics and Elixirs

Tonics and *elixirs* are similar to tinctures because they are made with alcohol.

The only difference between a tonic and a tincture is that a *tonic* is a blend of herbs formulated for long-term use to bring some aspect of the body back into balance. An example of this is the Concentration Tonic (page 110), a blend of different herbs that are supportive and restorative to the nervous system with a focus on the brain.

Elixirs are made just like tinctures, with the addition of honey to sweeten the formula. These are ideal for kids who may dislike the tincture taste. An example of an *elixir* is the Chickenpox Elixir (page 126).

To make an elixir: *Mix 1 part honey with 4 to 8 parts tincture. (For instance, in the Chickenpox Elixir [page 126], you mix 3½ ounces tincture with ½ ounce honey.) It is helpful to gently heat your honey first so that it's thin and pourable, then add it to the jar with the tincture and shake to combine.*

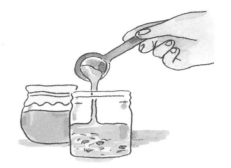

I prefer to use local honey to take advantage of pollen from the surrounding area, which helps boost the body's immune system against local allergens. The honey in elixirs is usually added after the blend is formulated, but if you are making a single elixir, you can add honey when you tincture the herb.

For instance, to make a wild cherry elixir, follow the instructions for making a tincture (page 63), measure the amount of tincture you have, and then add up to ¼ that amount of honey to the jar. For an 8-ounce tincture, you would add 1 to 2 ounces of honey.

A great example of a combined tonic and elixir is the Immune System Boost & Support Tonic Elixir (page 132). This formula can be taken long term to help boost the immune system. It's also sweetened with honey, so kids won't grumble about taking it on a daily basis.

Oils

Herb-infused *oils* (or *oil infusions*) are not the same as essential oils. Essential oils are specific medicinal constituents that are extracted from an herb, making a very potent and concentrated oil—and one that can be toxic if used improperly.

An oil infusion is similar to a tea. When you heat the oil with herbs in it, the heat helps to extract their medicinal properties. It's best to use dried herbs, though freshly wilted herbs can work, too. Just make sure to let the completed, strained oil sit for 24 hours so any residual moisture will sink to the bottom and the oil can be poured off.

∿ STORAGE ∾

How you store your herbs is just as important as where you source them. And if you've grown them yourself and taken the time to carefully dry them, the last thing you want is for them to go bad because of improper storage.

There are several ways to store herbs. I like to store mine in glass jars in a cabinet. Each glass jar is airtight and labeled with the common and the botanical names of the plant, the part of the plant that was harvested for the remedy, the date and location of where it was harvested, and any other pertinent information. For instance, I like to harvest New England aster flowers midday when the sun is at its peak and they are most sticky with resin, so I add the time to my label. If you have purchased your herbs, note where you purchased them, the date they were purchased, and the lot number (if the package has one).

My friend Rebekah likes to reuse cardboard oatmeal containers for storing herbs because they are fairly airtight and don't let light in.

Paper bags also can work well to store herbs, especially bark. Place your dried herbs in the bag, roll the lip closed, and use a rubber band to secure the bag. Don't forget a label.

No matter your storage choice, keep herbs out of direct light and in a cool location. I have a large sideboard with cabinet doors. In a perfect world, my herbs would be alphabetized, but because the jars vary, I store them according to size. On my computer, I list my herbs by shelf so I can do a word search to quickly find the location of each one.

You can use any type of oil. Coconut oil and olive oil are two good all-purpose oils that are on the greasy side, allowing the infusion to sit on the skin longer before being absorbed. Sweet almond oil and jojoba oil are lighter oils that are great for massaging and facial applications. Hemp seed oil is highly nutritious, full of antioxidants, protein, carotene, phytosterols, and many vitamins and minerals. Castor oil is an extremely thick oil that is great for drawing out toxins from the skin.

Oil can be used externally or internally. *Infused oils* make great salad dressing oils. Oils also can be blended into creams, lotions, salves, and lip balms.

To make an infused oil: *Combine ½ cup of dried herbs and 1½ cups of oil. Use one of the following methods to infuse your oil.*

Solar infusion: Combine the herbs and oil in a jar, screw on the lid, and set the jar in the sun for about 2 weeks to heat the oil and infuse it with the herbs.

Slow cooker method: Combine the herbs and oil in a mini slow cooker, cover, and heat on the Warm setting for 8 to 24 hours. If necessary, use intermittent heat by turning the slow cooker off and back on throughout the day to keep the oil from boiling.

Double boiler method: Fill the bottom of a double boiler or a medium saucepan about ⅓ with water and bring it to a simmer over medium-low heat. Place the herbs and oil in the top of a double boiler or in a bowl or glass measuring cup, and set it in the saucepan so the bottom of the pan, bowl, or measuring cup hovers above the simmering water. Heat the herb-oil mixture gently for 8 to 24 hours. Do not leave the stove unattended; turn off the heat overnight, and cover the herb-oil mixture with a lid for longer heating times.

Once the herbs have been infused into the oil, line a fine-mesh strainer with cheesecloth or other light fabric and pour the herbs through the strainer into a jar or other airtight container. Let the oil drip through the fabric, and do not squeeze the herbs and oil because this can introduce moisture into the oil.

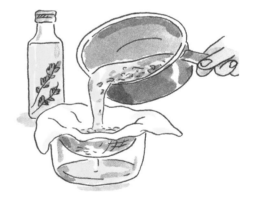

When all the oil has dripped into the jar, empty a vitamin E gelcap into your oil to help preserve it. Seal the jar and store it in the refrigerator. Be sure to label the jar with the type of oil and date infused. Oils last for about 1 year in the fridge.

Note: No matter which infusion method you use, NEVER let the oil boil. It will fry the herbs and make the infused oil worthless. It's better to heat the oil to just before boiling, turn off the heat, and let it cool before repeating, rather than risk overheating the oil.

Salves

Herbal *salves* are herb-infused oils that have been thickened with beeswax or other wax, such as candelilla. Lip balms are basically herbal salves. For a good lip balm recipe, see the Fever Blister Lip Balm recipe (page 218) in chapter 10. You can swap in your infused oils to make any blend of lip balm.

Salves are a little less messier than oils, since they tend to stay where you apply them, and they can be used for a variety of purposes. There are several salve recipes in this book, including Bruise and Bump Salve (page 83), Cuts and Scrapes Salve (page 86), and Plantar Fasciitis Salve (page 193). Salves can help disinfect, heal, and relieve wounds and pain.

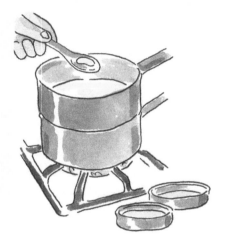

To make a salve: *Fill the bottom of a double boiler or a medium saucepan about ⅓ full with water and bring it to a simmer over medium-low heat. In the top of a double boiler or in a bowl or glass measuring cup, combine 1 part wax for every 8 parts oil (for example, 1 ounce wax and 8 ounces oil). Set the top of the double boiler (or bowl or measuring cup) in the saucepan so the bottom of the pan, bowl, or measuring cup hovers above the simmering water. Heat the mixture until the wax melts. Once the wax has melted completely, scoop up a few drops with a spoon, let it cool, and then test the consistency with your finger. If it's too soft, add more wax. If it's too firm, add more oil. Keep in mind that the salve will firm up a bit more in its container than it will on the spoon.*

When you are happy with the consistency, transfer the salve to an airtight tin or jar. You may wish to pour some salve into lip balm tubes. They can be tucked into your purse, briefcase, backpack, or everyday carry bag for relief on the go.

Salves can be stored for about 6 months to 1 year. You'll know when they are bad because they'll smell rancid. As with all preparations, make a habit of sniffing salves every time you open them up so you are familiar with their normal scents and can tell when they have expired.

Syrups

Syrups are a great way to get kids to take their medicine, especially for soothing sore throats and coughs. Syrups are fairly easy to make. Just brew an herbal infusion, then slowly thicken it by adding honey or sugar.

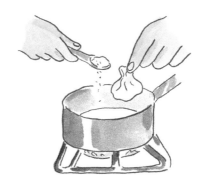

To make syrup: *Start with a strong tea. In a medium saucepan, combine ½ cup of dried herbs and 16 ounces of water. I like to put my herbs in a tea ball or muslin bag to help make straining easy. Bring the water to a boil, then turn off the heat, cover the pan, and let the mixture steep for 15 to 30 minutes. Strain the tea through a fine-mesh sieve into a large measuring cup. Note the volume of strained tea, and measure half of that amount of sugar into a saucepan*. Pour the strained tea into the saucepan with the sugar, place the pan over medium-low heat, and cook it until the liquid has reduced by half. Do not let your tea boil; you want to slowly evaporate the water.*

> **In the Cough Soother Syrup (page 86), for example, you'll have 16 ounces of tea. Add 8 ounces of sugar to the pan and cook down to 16 ounces total. If you are adding honey instead of sugar, there's no need to cook down the formula. Simply add the same amount of honey (in this case, 8 ounces), and stir to dissolve it into the tea. Store your syrup in an airtight jar in the fridge, where it will generally last for about 3 to 6 months.*

Creams and Lotions

Creams and *lotions* are basically salves that have added water and need to be blended together with a hand mixer or whisk—a process that can be a bit tricky, since oil and water don't like to mix. Patience, persistence, and a bit of borax help make smooth, emulsified products.

Creams are typically heavier than lotions and contain less water than lotions. *Creams* tend to feel stickier than lotions and are more moisturizing. *Lotions* are less sticky and more quickly absorbed into the skin. While lotion can be put into a pump bottle, creams are best stored in a wide-mouthed jar because they are too thick to pump. In this book, I focus on creams, including Arthritis and Gout Cream (page 177), Sun Care Cream (page 209), Scar Repair Cream (page 208), and Shaving Cream (page 204).

To make a cream (or lotion): *Fill the bottom of a double boiler or a medium saucepan about one-third full with water and bring it to a simmer over medium-low heat. In the top of a double boiler or in a bowl or glass measuring cup, combine the oils and wax. Set the top of the double boiler (or bowl or measuring cup) in the saucepan so the bottom of the pan, bowl, or measuring cup*

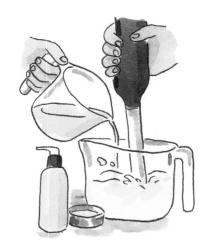

hovers above the simmering water. Heat the mixture until the wax melts, then remove the pan from the heat and pour the mixture into a 4-cup glass measuring cup; set aside to cool.

While the oils and wax are cooling, heat the water in a clean saucepan, add the herbs to make a tea, and then stir in the borax until it is completely dissolved. Remove the pan from the heat and set it aside to cool.

Once the oils and tea are both at room temperature, begin mixing the oil with a stick blender. Slowly start drizzling the tea into the oil, a little at a time, blending continuously. The mixture will begin to take on a creamy appearance. Once you have combined the oils and tea, stop blending and pour the mixture into a wide-mouth jar. Seal the jar and store your cream in a cool location. Creams and lotions typically last for up to 1 year.

➹ LABELING HERBS AND HOMEMADE REMEDIES ➷

If there's one mantra I want you to remember, it's "Label, label, label!" It's really important to label all your herbs and remedies! Dried herbs and tinctures tend to look the same when they are in unlabeled jars, and it can be dangerous to assume the identity of an herb or remedy. It doesn't have to be fancy—a piece of paper taped to the jar works fine. Use a waterproof pen or marker on any label, and cover the entire label with clear packing tape for extra protection.

What should be on a label?

If it's a single herb, label it with the common and botanical name of the herb, when/where it was harvested (or, if purchased, where it was purchased and when along with a lot number, if applicable). For tea blends, write down all the herbs in the tea, when it was made, its use, and how to use it.

If it's a formula, list out all the ingredients, add the date it was made, and describe how to use the remedy. For a tincture, write down the common and botanical names of the herb, the date it was started, the proportions of plant to menstruum, and the amount of and type of alcohol.

Oils, salves, creams, lotions, and syrups should all have similar labels that list the ingredients, dates made, and instructions.

Compresses, Poultices, and Plasters

Compresses also are known as *fomentations*. Typically, they are made using a diffusion or decoction of an herb and a soft cloth such as flannel. The infusion (temperature of the compress) can be either hot or cold. Alternatively, full-strength or diluted tinctures can be applied in place of infusions or decoctions. The Sprains and Strains Compress (page 101), is a good example.

> **To make a compress:** *Soak a soft cloth in the diffusion or decoction. Gently squeeze out the excess liquid, then apply the cloth to the injured area of the body. Reapply as the compress cools or warms to room temperature.*

Poultices are made from fresh or dried herbs. They can be simple, such as a spit poultice, which is a fresh herb chewed up and spit out (or chopped and broken down with hot water) and placed on the wound.

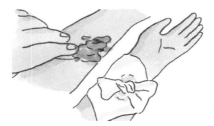

To make a poultice: *Either chew the herbs or chop and steep them in hot water. After the herbs have steeped for a few minutes, strain off the liquid and apply the herbs directly to the skin. Cover them with a soft cloth such as flannel, and bind them to the body with a stretch bandage. Leave the poultice on for several hours or overnight. Reapply once or twice a day.*

The Bee Sting Poultice (page 81), Spider Bite Poultice (page 99), and Splinter Poultice (page 100) are great (and easy-to-make) examples of poultices.

Plasters, which typically are used for congestion and respiratory complaints, consist of dried, powdered herb combined with cornmeal or flour.

To make a plaster: *Mix together equal parts of the herb and flour, and moisten with water, herbal tea, or tincture. Spread the paste on a flannel cloth, and place the flannel cloth over the wound site.*

Tip: To help heat compresses, poultices, and plasters, press a hot water bottle on top when you apply it directly to your body.

Powders

Powders are herbs that have been finely ground. The herbs can be mixed with other powders such as arrowroot, flour, or cornstarch or with clays such as bentonite, French, and kaolin. They are great for applying dry to a weeping wound (see Nosebleed Powder on page 137) or helping dry out delicate areas of the body (see Chafing Powder on page 167).

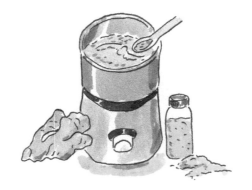

Tinctures and teas, or even water, can be added to powders to make plasters that will adhere to the skin. You can also use powders to make Energy Balls (page 182), and you can mix powder with a few drops of honey to make tasty "pills" that are especially appealing to kids.

You can buy herbs already powdered or use a coffee grinder to make your own. (Be sure to buy one dedicated to grinding medicinal herbs.) After grinding, sift powders through a fine-mesh strainer. A mortar and pestle also can be used to grind down herbs, though it can take a lot longer when working with harder parts such as roots and barks.

Baths

Ahhhh, baths! Who doesn't love a good, relaxing bath? Did you know that a bath can be a great way to get a dose of herbs? Bath teas can be made to treat a variety of ailments, from fevers to achy muscles and nervous tension. *Herbal baths* help open the pores of the skin, your largest organ, making it easy for your body to absorb the herbs' medicinal properties.

To make an herbal bath: *Use 3 to 4 ounces of a single herb or blend. Heat a stockpot full of water, place the herbs in a cheesecloth tied with a rubber band, and steep for about 30 minutes. Pour the diffusion into your bath water, and soak for 20 to 30 minutes.*

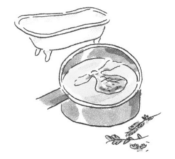

Hotter baths can be helpful for sore, achy muscles. Take the Sore Muscle Salve (page 98) herbs, turn them into a tea blend, and you've got a great herbal bath tea!

A warm water bath is more soothing for nerves. A simple oatmeal bath or the Nerve Pain Relief Tea Blend (page 95) work great for this application.

Cooler or tepid water is better for fevers. Try the Fever-Reducing Popsicles (page 130) as a bath soak if your child doesn't want to eat Popsicles or drink a cup of tea. (Also, see chapter 10 for a great basic bath tea recipe, Bath Tea Blend, on page 203.)

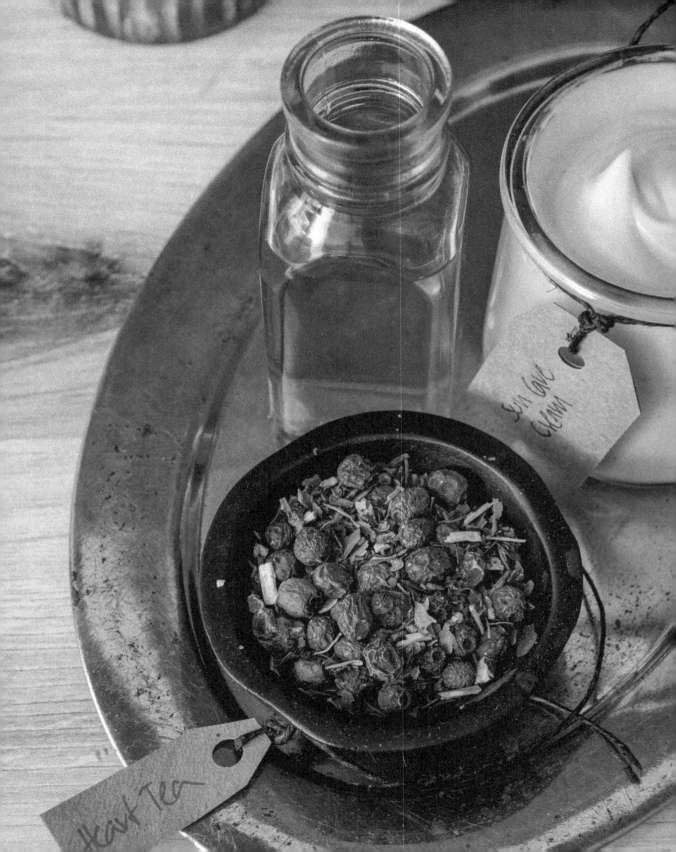

PART TWO

RECIPES

Now that you've learned all about these herbs and how to use them, let's jump into the recipes!

Part 2 is divided into seven chapters with 125 recipes total. Each chapter focuses on a topic to help you narrow your search.

In chapter 4, you'll find recipes to help with minor injuries like bumps, bruises, and scrapes. Chapter 5 offers a variety of recipes to remedy mental health conditions, including depression, insomnia, and stress. If you have kids, you'll probably spend a lot of time in chapter 6, where you'll find a variety of recipes for treating everything from nightmares to fevers. Chapters 7 and 8 focus on the specific needs of adult women and men, and chapter 9 offers help for aging issues, including acid reflux and heart health. Finally, chapter 10 offers ideas for healthy skin, mouth, and hair.

As a reminder, please be sure to review the safety considerations for each herb before use.

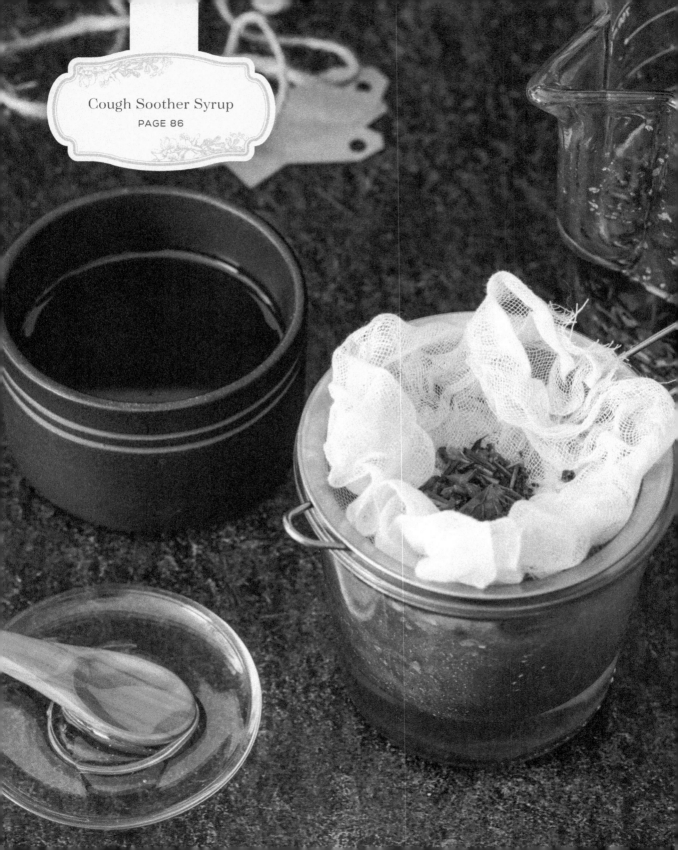

Cough Soother Syrup
PAGE 86

CHAPTER FOUR

COMMON AILMENTS

In this chapter, you'll find more than 25 recipes to help you with everyday ailments, from little bumps and scrapes to splinters, tick and spider bites, and bee stings. You'll learn how to use herbs with poultices, compresses, formulas, and teas to make you feel better, faster.

We'll also dive into remedies for colds and the flu, as well as digestive issues such as diarrhea and constipation, indigestion and gas, leaky gut, irritable bowel syndrome, and nausea. And since no one enjoys muscle pain, there are a variety of recipes to ease muscle spasms, sprains, and strains, as well as sore muscles from overexertion at the gym.

Finally, there are recipes for other common ailments such as ringworm and nerve pain.

ALLERGY RELIEF FORMULA

Itchy eyes, a scratchy throat, and constant sneezing are frequent symptoms of seasonal allergies. This blend boosts the body's histamine response and provides relief. It also is helpful for pet dander and other allergies.

1. Add tinctures to a 1-cup glass measuring cup and stir to combine.

2. Pour the mixture into an 8-ounce glass dropper bottle. Tighten the dropper lid on the bottle, then label with the list of ingredients, date, and instructions for use.

TO USE: Add 40 to 60 drops of tincture to a small glass of water or juice and drink 3 times daily. During an acute allergy episode, you may wish to take the standard dose every 15 minutes for 1 to 2 hours to help boost your body's response to the allergens. Continue with the normal dose for the rest of the day.

NOTE: This formula also can be blended as a tea. For more allergy relief, consider drinking 1 to 2 cups of infusion of stinging nettles several times a week throughout the year to help reduce the histamine reaction. This recipe can be doubled, tripled, etc.

Makes 8 ounces

3 ounces goldenrod tincture

2 ounces stinging nettle leaf tincture

1½ ounces New England aster tincture

1½ ounces plantain tincture

ASTHMA FORMULA

Asthma can damage lung tissue. Take this formula at the first inkling of an asthma attack for best results. The combination of herbs helps to relieve lung spasms while relaxing the bronchial tubes.

1. Add the tinctures to a 1-cup glass measuring cup and stir to combine.

2. Pour the mixture into an 8-ounce glass dropper bottle.

3. Tighten the dropper lid on the bottle, then label with the list of ingredients, date, and instructions for use.

Makes 8 ounces

4 ounces New England aster tincture

2 ounces wild cherry bark tincture

2 ounces wild lettuce leaf tincture

TO USE: Add 30 to 60 drops of tincture to a small glass of water or juice and drink 3 times daily. During an acute asthma episode, you may wish to take 60 drops every 10 to 15 minutes until your lungs begin to relax. Reduce the frequency to every 20 minutes until you are feeling relaxed. Continue with the normal dose for the rest of the day.

NOTE: Be sure to support your lungs by drinking herbal infusions such as stinging nettles, milky oats, and plantain several times a week in addition to taking this formula as suggested.

BEE STING POULTICE

Remove the stinger before using this remedy. Plantain helps to draw out the venom, soothes the inflammation, and eases pain. Wild cherry helps cool the inflammation.

For best results, chew the plantain leaves until they are mashed into a poultice. This provides saliva, which has healing properties. (Alternatively, the leaves can be finely chopped and mixed with a bit of boiling water. Steep for 15 minutes, then strain.)

TO USE: Mix the plantain with the tincture, then place the mixture place directly on the bite. Gently wipe off, and repeat every 20 to 30 minutes until the swelling has receded.

NOTE: Flexible bandage wraps can be helpful for holding the poultice in place. If the poultice heats up and the sting site is still quite red, swollen, and painful, the poultice can be replaced more frequently. For best results, follow up the poultice by drinking a cup of water with 60 drops each of plantain and wild cherry tincture.

Makes 1 poultice

- 1 to 2 fresh plantain leaves or 1 teaspoon dried plantain
- 30 drops wild cherry tincture
- 1 tablespoon boiling water (optional)

BRONCHITIS FORMULA

This formula, along with a nourishing diet and plenty of bed rest, should be enough to clear up acute bronchitis. If you do not show signs of improvement after 2 days, follow up with your medical or herbal practitioner.

1. Add the tinctures to a 1-cup glass measuring cup and stir to combine.

2. Pour the mixture into an 8-ounce glass dropper bottle.

3. Tighten the dropper lid on the bottle, then label with the list of ingredients, date, and instructions for use.

TO USE: At the first sign of symptoms, add 30 drops of tincture to a small glass of water or juice. Repeat hourly for 4 hours, then decrease to every 2 hours for the first day. Take every 4 hours on the second day and every 6 hours on the third day. Continue taking 3 times daily until all symptoms have cleared.

NOTE: For chronic bronchitis, add herbal infusions such as stinging nettles, milky oats, and plantain several times a week to your routine to strengthen the lungs while taking this formula as suggested.

Makes 8 ounces

2½ ounces ground ivy tincture

2 ounces spilanthes tincture

2 ounces New England aster tincture

1½ ounces wild lettuce tincture

BRUISE AND BUMP SALVE

Keep this salve on hand for the little bumps and bruises. These herbs can help soothe pain and break down stagnant blood to more quickly heal bruising.

1. Follow the instructions on page 68 to make a salve.

2. Label with the list of ingredients, date, and instructions for use.

TO USE: To use, apply a small amount of salve to bumps, blows, and bruises. Reapply every 4 to 6 hours as needed.

NOTE: Pour salve into a lip balm tube to use on the go.

Makes 4 ounces

1½ ounces prunella-infused oil

1 ounce gotu kola–infused oil

1 ounce yarrow-infused oil

½ ounce beeswax

1 vitamin E gelcap

BURN CARE WRAP

Burdock leaf has been shown to be an effective burn healer. I've seen its power to heal a burn firsthand. If you don't have St. John's wort tincture, you can substitute gotu kola tincture or omit the tincture altogether. Burdock leaf works well enough on its own.

1. If the leaf is fresh, roll it with a rolling pin. Place the leaf into a pot of boiling water for 30 seconds.

2. Pull the leaf out of the boiling water with tongs and let it cool. You also may plunge the leaf into ice water to cool it more quickly.

3. Cut off a portion of the leaf that is big enough to wrap around the burn.

Makes 3 to 4 wraps

1 burdock leaf
10 drops St. John's wort tincture

TO USE: Apply the St. John's wort tincture directly to the burn, then wrap the cooled leaf over the burn. When the leaf gets warm, remove it and repeat the process with a fresh piece of blanched and cooled leaf. Once the leaf remains cool on the burn, wrap it with a self-adhesive elastic bandage to hold it in place. Check and replace the burdock leaf every 8 to 12 hours until the burn has healed.

NOTE: Before applying the herbs, be sure to hold the burn in cool water for several minutes to help reduce the burn. Do not use ice water. For severe burns, seek medical assistance.

COLD CARE TEA BLEND

Brew a cup of this tea anytime you feel a cold coming on. It can help prevent a cold from setting in or offer relief if you've already come down with something.

Combine all the ingredients, and store in an airtight container. Label the container with the list of ingredients, date, and instructions for use.

TO USE: Steep 2 teaspoons of the tea blend in 8 ounces of boiling water for 15 to 20 minutes.

NOTE: You may wish to add 30 drops of monarda tincture to the tea for an extra boost.

Makes enough for 25 cups of tea

½ cup dried prunella

¼ cup dried ground ivy

2 tablespoons dried monarda

2 tablespoons dried yarrow

1 tablespoon dried spearmint

CONSTIPATION-FREE TEA BLEND

Drinking 1 to 2 cups of this tea a day will help keep you regular. Be sure to include enough water in your daily diet, since constipation is often a sign of dehydration.

Combine all the ingredients, and store in an airtight container. Label the container with the list of ingredients, date, and instructions for use.

TO USE: Bring 12 ounces of water to a boil with 1 tablespoon of tea blend. Simmer for 15 to 20 minutes. Drink 2 to 3 cups daily.

NOTE: A bit of honey and some almond or oat milk can be added to help sweeten this tea.

Makes enough for 16 cups of tea

½ cup dried burdock root

½ cup dried dandelion root

½ cup dried yellow dock root

¼ cup dried ginger

¼ cup dried catnip

COUGH SOOTHER SYRUP

This blend of herbs helps break up and dry out mucus, kills cough-causing germs, and soothes irritated bronchial tubes.

1. Follow the instructions on page 69 to make a syrup.

2. Transfer the syrup to an airtight jar or bottle. Screw on the lid, then label with the list of ingredients, date, and instructions for use.

3. Store in the refrigerator. Use within 3 months.

TO USE: Take 1 to 3 teaspoons as needed to help ease coughs and soothe sore throats.

NOTE: Try adding more honey to sweeten this syrup, up to 16 ounces.

Makes 24 ounces

¼ cup dried wild cherry

2 tablespoons dried prunella

1 tablespoon dried ground ivy

2 teaspoons dried thyme

1 teaspoon dried wild lettuce

16 ounces water

8 ounces honey

CUTS AND SCRAPES SALVE

This salve is a great multipurpose remedy for cuts and scrapes. Calendula helps keep the cut infection free, while plantain and yarrow help quickly stop bleeding. Prunella and gotu kola help heal the wound.

1. Follow the instructions on page 68 to make a salve.

2. Label with the list of ingredients, date, and instructions for use.

TO USE: Apply as needed to cuts and scrapes.

NOTE: This recipe can be made into a tea blend to be used as a wash on wounds as well as powdered to sprinkle on weepy wounds and help them dry.

Makes 4 ounces

1 ounce gotu kola–infused oil

1 ounce calendula-infused oil

½ ounce plantain-infused oil

½ ounce prunella-infused oil

½ ounce yarrow-infused oil

½ ounce beeswax

1 vitamin E gelcap

DIARRHEA RELIEF FORMULA

This formula can be helpful for relieving diarrhea and related dehydration. Follow up with an electrolyte drink to help replenish fluids. Be sure to seek medical assistance to find out the cause, especially in the case of chronic diarrhea.

1. Add the tinctures to a 1-cup glass measuring cup and stir to combine.

2. Pour the mixture into a 2-ounce glass dropper bottle.

3. Tighten the dropper lid on the bottle, then label with the list of ingredients, date, and instructions for use.

TO USE: Add 30 drops of tincture to a small glass of water or juice, and drink every 15 minutes until the diarrhea subsides. Take every 30 minutes for 1 hour.

NOTE: Be sure to rehydrate the body with fluids. A natural electrolyte drink can be made with 8 ounces water, 1 tablespoon fresh lemon juice, 1 tablespoon honey, and 1 pinch sea salt.

Makes 2 ounces

1 ounce blackberry root tincture
1 ounce catnip tincture

ECZEMA AND PSORIASIS SUPPORT FORMULA

Eczema and psoriasis often result from liver issues. Toning herbs such as burdock and dandelion help support the liver, while yellow dock eases inflammation.

1. Add the tinctures to a 1-cup glass measuring cup and stir to combine.

2. Pour the mixture into a 4-ounce glass dropper bottle.

3. Tighten the dropper lid on the bottle, then label with the list of ingredients, date, and instructions for use.

Makes 4 ounces

2 ounces burdock root tincture

1 ounce dandelion root tincture

1 ounce yellow dock tincture

TO USE: Add 30 to 60 drops of tincture to a small glass of water or juice, and drink 3 times daily.

NOTE: Limit your consumption of sugar, caffeine, and processed foods while trying to support and heal the liver.

HEADACHE RELIEF TEA BLEND

Headaches can be caused by many different things: stress, digestive issues, and tension, to name a few. In this spicy and pungent all-purpose blend, ginger helps increase circulation to the brain, while black haw and wild lettuce help reduce pain and relax tension.

Combine the ingredients, and store in an airtight container. Label with the list of ingredients, date, and instructions for use.

Makes enough for 25 cups of tea

½ cup dried ginger
¼ cup dried black haw
¼ cup dried wild lettuce

TO USE: Steep 2 teaspoons of the tea blend in 8 ounces of boiling water for 15 to 20 minutes. Drink 1 to 2 cups to ease the headache.

NOTE: This blend also can be made into a tincture and taken 30 drops every 15 to 20 minutes as needed.

INDIGESTION AND GAS TEA BLEND

Sip this tea to help with gas and indigestion. If acid reflux is a regular problem for you, see the Acid Reflux Formula on page 175. This blend is spicy with a hint of mint. The rosemary, thyme, and mugwort flavors balance out the mint and ginger without being too overwhelming.

Combine all the ingredients, and store in an air-tight container. Label with the list of ingredients, date, and instructions for use.

TO USE: Steep 2 teaspoons of the tea blend in 8 ounces of boiling water for 15 to 20 minutes. Drink 1 to 2 cups after a meal, as needed.

NOTE: To help encourage intestinal movement, lie down on your back and gently stroke your abdomen in a large, circular clockwise motion.

Makes enough for 25 cups of tea

¼ cup dried spearmint

¼ cup dried ginger

3 tablespoons dried rosemary

3 tablespoons dried thyme

2 tablespoons dried mugwort

INFLUENZA CARE FORMULA

Start taking this formula at the first sign of the flu. These herbs work great to help the body fight off germs from influenza, reduce fever, and ease aches and pains. Prunella fights the influenza virus, while goldenrod eases aches and pains. Yarrow helps reduce fevers and is antiviral, mugwort eases general malaise and digestive issues, and spearmint eases fever, pain, and nausea.

1. Add the tinctures to a 1-cup glass measuring cup and stir to combine.

2. Pour the mixture into an 8-ounce glass dropper bottle.

3. Tighten the dropper lid on the bottle, then label with the list of ingredients, date, and instructions for use.

Makes 8 ounces

3 ounces prunella tincture
2 ounces goldenrod
  tincture
1 ounce yarrow tincture
1 ounce mugwort tincture
1 ounce spearmint tincture

TO USE: Add 30 to 60 drops of tincture to a small glass of water or juice and drink 4 to 6 times daily. This formula also can be used as a tea blend by steeping 1 tablespoon in 8 ounces of boiling water for 15 to 20 minutes. Consume every 1 to 2 hours as needed.

NOTE: You may also wish to add 30 drops of spilanthes tincture to each dose for extra immune support.

LEAKY GUT & IRRITABLE BOWEL TEA BLEND

Leaky gut is a general term for a range of symptoms indicating something is going on (often undiagnosed) in the digestive system, and Irritable Bowel Syndrome (IBS) is a disorder in the large intestine. Both present with similar symptoms: bloating, gas, cramping and abdominal pain, diarrhea, constipation, and food sensitivities. The herbs in this blend help support healthy digestion, heal intestinal inflammation, and soothe spasms. The tea is mild in flavor, with a bit of spiciness from the ginger and monarda and a hint of mint from the spearmint.

Combine all the ingredients, and store in an airtight container. Label with the list of ingredients, date, and instructions for use.

TO USE: Steep 1 tablespoon tea blend in 10 ounces of boiling water for 15 to 20 minutes. Drink 2 to 3 cups daily.

NOTE: It's important when trying to heal a leaky gut to follow a diet that removes offending foods such as wheat, corn, dairy, soy, sugar, and alcohol. When a proper diet is combined with this tea, you'll notice improvement. Consider having a health care professional test you for allergies, and follow their recommended elimination diet.

Makes enough for 30 cups of tea

½ cup dried plantain
¼ cup dried
   blackberry leaves
¼ cup dried ginger
¼ cup dried monarda
¼ cup dried spearmint
2 tablespoons dried black
   walnut leaves
2 tablespoons
   dried borage
2 tablespoons mugwort

MUSCLE SPASM OIL

These herbs are great for soothing muscle spasms. Use this infused oil blend for muscle cramps everywhere, from back pain to menstrual cramps and charley horses.

1. Combine the oils together in a glass measuring cup and stir to combine.

2. Pour into an 8-ounce bottle.

3. Tighten the lid on the bottle, then label with the list of ingredients, date, and instructions for use. Store in the refrigerator, and discard at the first sign of rancidity.

TO USE: Massage room-temperature or warmed oil into muscles and reapply as needed.

NOTE: You may also wish to make a tincture formula from this tea blend to take internally.

Makes 8 ounces

2 ounces mugwort-infused oil

2 ounces black haw–infused oil

2 ounces goldenrod-infused oil

2 ounces catnip-infused oil

NAUSEA RELIEF TEA BLEND

Nausea can be caused by a variety of issues from motion sickness to digestive upset to a virus. Ginger and spearmint are both very soothing to the stomach, helping to ease nausea. The flavor is familiar, sweet, and spicy.

Combine all the ingredients, and store in an airtight container. Label with the list of ingredients, date, and instructions for use.

Makes enough for 48 cups of tea

1 cup dried ginger
1 cup dried spearmint

TO USE: Steep 2 teaspoons of the tea blend in 8 ounces of boiling water for 15 to 20 minutes.

NOTE: Add a spoonful of honey to sweeten, if desired.

NERVE PAIN RELIEF TEA BLEND

This tea blend can ease nervous tension and nerve pain. Milky oats and St. John's wort are two herbs that specifically aid nervous system function. Black haw and wild lettuce help reduce pain and sedate the nervous system. Milky oats have a sweet, mild flavor that is balanced well with the bitterness of black haw and wild lettuce to make a well-rounded tea.

Combine all the ingredients, and store in an airtight container. Label with the list of ingredients, date, and instructions for use.

TO USE: Steep 1 tablespoon of the tea blend in 8 ounces of boiling water for 15 to 20 minutes. Drink 2 to 3 cups daily.

NOTE: It also may help to apply St. John's wort–infused oil or tincture topically to afflicted nerves, massaging as needed.

Makes enough for 32 cups of tea

1¼ cups dried milky oats
½ cup dried black haw
¼ cup dried wild lettuce

RINGWORM TOPICAL SOLUTION

Ringworm isn't actually a worm; it's a fungus that causes a patch of circular, red, raised skin. It may be itchy and scaly and requires antifungals to eliminate it and prevent it from spreading. Black walnut and monarda work effectively as antifungals to quickly reduce the itching, irritation, and scaliness, as well as the fungus. This topical solution can be applied to any kind of fungus with effective results.

1. Add the tinctures to a 1-cup glass measuring cup and stir to combine.

2. Pour the mixture into a 1-ounce glass dropper bottle.

3. Tighten the dropper lid on the bottle, then label with the list of ingredients, date, and instructions for use.

Makes 1 ounce

¾ ounce black walnut hull tincture
¼ ounce monarda tincture

TO USE: Apply several drops directly onto the ringworm site, and lightly massage. Repeat 1 to 2 times daily until the area is cleared up.

NOTE: Black walnut hull tincture can stain your skin. You may wish to use black walnut leaves instead if the fungus is in a visible location.

SINUS CONGESTION TEA BLEND

Painful pressure in the nasal cavities, behind the eyes, and along the jaw caused by congested sinuses can make you feel miserable, especially when your nasal tissues are inflamed, stuffy, and full of mucus. This combination of sinus herbs helps to soothe inflamed membranes, dry up mucus, and clear infection.

Combine all the ingredients, and store in an air-tight container. Label with the list of ingredients, date, and instructions for use.

TO USE: Steep 2 teaspoons of the tea blend in 8 ounces of boiling water for 15 to 20 minutes. Drink 1 to 2 cups as needed.

NOTE: ¼ teaspoon sea salt can be added to the tea to create a nasal wash for your neti pot to be used as needed. Follow the instructions from your neti pot for use.

Makes enough for 48 cups of tea

1 cup dried plantain
½ cup dried prunella
½ cup dried goldenrod

SORE MUSCLE SALVE

Whether you were working in a garden, doing heavy manual labor, or taking a hike up a mountain trail, your muscles can be sore after a long day of physical movement. Use this salve to soothe muscle pain and tenderness to make it easier to get out of bed the next day.

1. Follow the instructions on page 68 to make a salve.

2. Label with the list of ingredients, date, and instructions for use.

TO USE: Massage as needed into sore muscles.

NOTE: The beeswax and vitamin E oil can be omitted to make a massage oil blend. For extra relief, take a bath with goldenrod tea first, then massage the salve into your sore muscles.

Makes 4 ounces

1 ounce goldenrod-infused oil

1 ounce prunella-infused oil

½ ounce rosemary-infused oil

½ ounce catnip-infused oil

½ ounce black haw–infused oil

½ ounce beeswax

1 vitamin E gelcap

SPIDER BITE POULTICE

This is great for spider bites and other insect bites. If you suspect a venomous spider bite, seek medical attention.

1. For best results, chew the plantain leaves until they are mashed into a poultice. This provides saliva, which contains healing properties. If you do not want to chew the poultice, the leaves can be chopped finely and mixed with a tablespoon of boiling water, then strained after 15 minutes.

2. Mix the plantain with the tincture and charcoal.

Makes 1 poultice

1 to 2 fresh plantain leaves or 1 teaspoon dried plantain
30 drops spilanthes tincture
1 teaspoon activated charcoal

TO USE: Apply directly to the spider bite. Repeat every 20 to 30 minutes until the swelling has receded.

NOTE: For an extra boost, take 30 drops of spilanthes tincture internally every 20 to 30 minutes for the first 2 hours.

SPLINTER POULTICE

This poultice works wonders for pulling out all sorts of slivers and splinters. The longer they've been under the skin and the deeper they are, the longer it will take to remove the splinters. Some splinters will come out right away, within hours, while some may take a week or longer—the longest I've had to wait was a week.

1. For best results, chew the plantain leaves until they are mashed into a poultice. This provides saliva, which contains healing properties. If you do not want to chew the poultice, the leaves can be chopped finely and mixed with a tablespoon of boiling water, then strained after 15 minutes.

2. Mix the plantain with the tincture and charcoal.

Makes 1 poultice

1 to 2 fresh plantain leaves or 1 teaspoon dried plantain

30 drops prunella tincture

1 teaspoon activated charcoal

TO USE: Apply directly over the splinter. Cover with a Band-Aid and repeat every 8 to 12 hours until the splinter has come to the surface and can be removed with tweezers.

NOTE: You may find the splinter comes out quicker if you gently "milk" the area where the splinter is located, massaging from the furthest point of penetration to the surface point of penetration each time you wipe off the existing poultice.

SPRAINS AND STRAINS COMPRESS

Sprains (overstretched or torn ligaments) and strains (overstretched or torn muscles or tendons) are painful and can immobilize you for a few days to a week. This compress reduces inflammation and helps heal damage to muscles, joints, and ligaments, promoting a quicker recovery. Use it immediately after an injury to prevent your condition from worsening.

1. Combine the herbs in a bowl and stir to blend. Store in a half gallon jar, labeled with the list of ingredients, date, and instructions for use.

2. To make your compress, boil 1 quart of water.

3. Add ½ cup to a quart jar and pour boiling water to top off jar.

4. Let steep for 20 minutes. Strain off the herbs and compost.

TO USE: Soak a piece of cloth in the tea, gently squeeze to remove the excess, and apply it to the strained muscle. Leave on for 20 minutes. Repeat the application 2 to 3 times daily for up to 2 weeks.

NOTE: The tea can be reheated and used for up to 4 days. Be sure to store in the fridge between uses.

Makes 6 quarts of tea for compresses

1 cup dried blackberry leaves

1 cup dried yarrow

½ cup dried comfrey leaves

½ cup dried black haw

STOMACH ULCER FORMULA

Stomach ulcers, also known as peptic or gastric ulcers, are sores that can be found in the lining of your stomach, esophagus, or small intestine. This formula is helpful for gastrointestinal irritation due to ulcers and inflammation. Plantain, calendula, and prunella help heal the wound, while black haw relieves inflammation and pain. Yarrow also has anti-inflammatory and healing properties, and St. John's wort eases nerve pain.

1. Add the tinctures to a 1-cup glass measuring cup and stir to combine.

2. Pour the mixture into a 4-ounce glass dropper bottle.

3. Tighten the dropper lid on the bottle, then label with the list of ingredients, date, and instructions for use.

Makes 4 ounces

1 ounce plantain tincture
1 ounce black haw tincture
½ ounce calendula tincture
½ ounce prunella tincture
½ ounce St. John's wort tincture
½ ounce yarrow tincture

TO USE: Add 20 to 40 drops of tincture to a small glass of water or juice and drink 3 times daily. For acute episodes, increase to 4 to 5 times daily.

NOTE: For best results, take along with the Leaky Gut & Irritable Bowel Tea Blend (page 92).

SWOLLEN LYMPH DRAIN FORMULA

Swollen lymph nodes can be very painful. Lymph is the body's way of clearing infection from the body. These herbs help clear the lymph after it has done its job.

1. Add the tinctures to a 1-cup glass measuring cup and stir to combine.

2. Pour the mixture into a 4-ounce glass dropper bottle.

3. Tighten the dropper lid on the bottle, then label with the list of ingredients, date, and instructions for use.

Makes 4 ounces

2 ounces cleavers tincture
1¾ ounces gotu kola
   tincture
¼ ounce poke root tincture

TO USE: Add 30 drops of tincture to a small glass of water or juice and drink 3 times daily until the lymph nodes have reduced in swelling.

NOTE: Lymph cannot move on its own. You might find movement such as jumping jacks to be helpful to help move the lymph, since the body has no pump for the lymph system like it does for the circulatory system.

TICK BITE FORMULA

If you suspect Lyme from a tick bite, this formula can help kill off the parasites that cause Lyme. Though it's best to seek medical attention for Lyme, it never hurts to take extra precautions.

1. Add the tinctures to a 1-cup glass measuring cup and stir to combine.

2. Pour the mixture into an 8-ounce glass dropper bottle.

3. Tighten the dropper lid on the bottle, then label with the list of ingredients, date, and instructions for use.

Makes 8 ounces

4 ounces spilanthes tincture
2 ounces plantain tincture
1 ounce mugwort tincture
1 ounce wild cherry tincture

TO USE: Add 30 to 60 drops of tincture to a small glass of water or juice and drink 3 times daily for at least 7 days and increase to 90 days if you suspect Lyme.

NOTE: Be diligent about checking for and removing ticks after being outdoors. When you are outdoors in a location that has ticks, wear clothing that is tight around the ankles and wrists to help prevent ticks from getting to your skin.

VERTIGO TAMER FORMULA

These three herbs excel at helping quell acute vertigo. If you are suffering from chronic vertigo, this formula can help relieve an attack, but for permanent relief, work to find the cause of the condition.

1. Add the tinctures to a 1-cup glass measuring cup and stir to combine.

2. Pour the tincture into a 4-ounce glass dropper bottle.

3. Tighten the dropper lid on the bottle, then label with the list of ingredients, date, and instructions for use.

TO USE: Add 30 drops of tincture to a small glass of water or juice and drink 3 times daily. For an acute episode, take 30 drops every 20 minutes as needed.

NOTE: Vertigo can be caused by many things. Be sure to drink plenty of fluids, get plenty of rest, avoid alcohol, and ask your health care practitioner about exercises that are best suited for your type of vertigo.

Makes 4 ounces

1½ ounces ginger tincture

1½ ounces ground ivy tincture

1 ounce monarda tincture

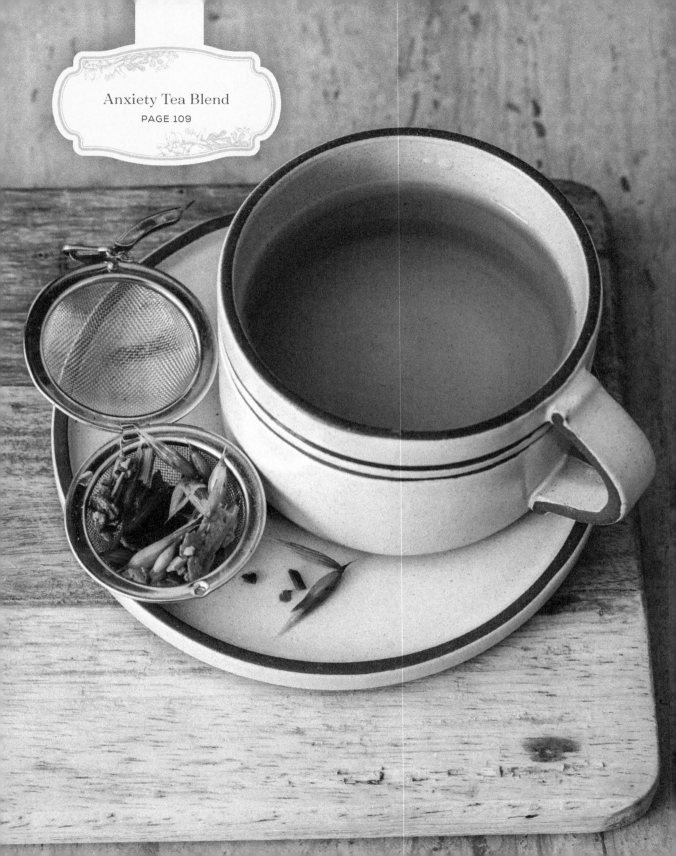

Anxiety Tea Blend

PAGE 109

CHAPTER FIVE

EMOTIONAL WELL-BEING

The everyday ups and downs of life can affect your well-being in subtle and not-so-subtle ways. Be sure to get plenty of rest, exercise, and wholesome foods for optimal emotional health. The recipes in this chapter are designed to help bolster emotional health by supporting the particular body systems that impact it—the nervous system, the cardiovascular system, and the endocrine system.

In this section, you'll find blends for anxiety, mental strain, general stress, and depression, as well as blends for heartbreak, fatigue, and insomnia.

These recipes are like your own personal cheering squad, working on the sidelines to support your body and mind when you need it most.

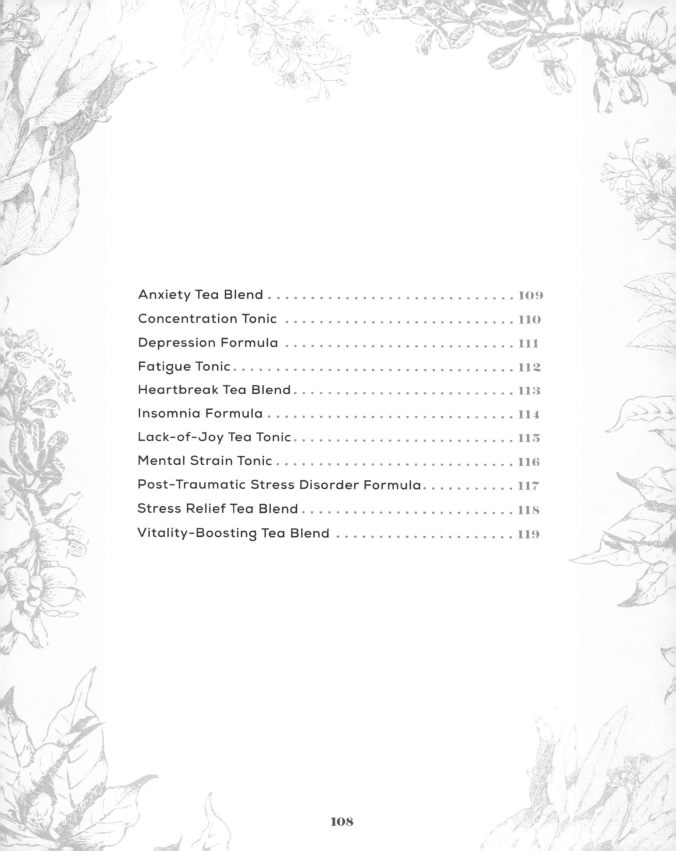

ANXIETY TEA BLEND

This blend of herbs is soothing to the nervous system, helping to calm and relax the mind. Though reishi is best extracted in a decoction, the longer steep time here helps draw out reishi's properties into the tea.

Combine all the ingredients, and store in an airtight container. Label with the list of ingredients, date, and instructions for use.

TO USE: Steep 1 tablespoon tea blend in 8 ounces of boiling water for 25 to 30 minutes. Drink 2 to 3 cups daily. Add a bit of honey if desired to sweeten.

NOTE: For an extra boost, add 30 drops of reishi tincture (page 34) to your cup of tea.

Makes enough for 32 cups of tea

1½ cups dried milky oats

3 tablespoons dried reishi

3 tablespoons dried wild cherry

2 tablespoons dried motherwort

CONCENTRATION TONIC

Difficulty concentrating can be caused by many things, including depression, stress, anxiety, fatigue, and hormonal changes. This tonic restores and supports the nervous system, stimulates the brain, aids in concentration, and helps you remain clear-headed.

1. Add the tinctures to a 1-cup glass measuring cup and stir to combine.

2. Pour the mixture into an 8-ounce glass dropper bottle.

3. Tighten the dropper lid on the bottle, then label with the list of ingredients, date, and instructions for use.

Makes 8 ounces

4 ounces gotu kola tincture

2 ounces rosemary tincture

1 ounce catnip tincture

½ ounce hawthorn berry tincture

½ ounce wild cherry tincture

TO USE: Add 20 to 40 drops of tincture to a small glass of water or juice and drink 3 times daily. For acute episodes, increase to 4 to 5 times daily.

NOTE: If you're having problems concentrating during a long work day, try to take a mini break every 1½ hours. Take a dose of the formula, get up and stretch, walk a few laps around the office to stretch your legs, and drink a glass of water. You should be ready to go when you sit back down.

DEPRESSION FORMULA

This formula is designed to support your nervous system and uplift your mood. If you suffer from seasonal affective disorder (SAD), try to get outside and take a good vitamin D_3 supplement daily.

1. Add the tinctures to a 1-cup glass measuring cup and stir to combine.

2. Pour the mixture into an 8-ounce glass dropper bottle.

3. Tighten the dropper lid on the bottle, then label with the list of ingredients, date, and instructions for use.

TO USE: Add 30 to 40 drops of tincture to a small glass of water or juice and drink 3 times daily. For acute episodes, increase to 4 to 5 times daily.

NOTE: You also can make this into a tea blend and substitute 30 drops of St. John's wort tincture in lieu of the actual herb in the tea.

Makes 8 ounces

3 ounces lemon balm tincture
1½ ounces goldenrod tincture
1½ ounces motherwort tincture
1 ounce hawthorn tincture
½ ounce mugwort tincture
½ ounce St. John's wort tincture

FATIGUE TONIC

This formula supports the endocrine system, liver, and nervous system while helping increase energy. Be sure to get plenty of rest, water, exercise, and wholesome foods to help replenish your energy as well. And make time to do the things you enjoy on a regular basis.

1. Add the tinctures to a 1-cup glass measuring cup and stir to combine.

2. Pour the mixture into an 8-ounce glass dropper bottle.

3. Tighten the dropper lid on the bottle, then label with the list of ingredients, date, and instructions for use.

TO USE: Add 30 to 40 drops of tincture to a small glass of water or juice and drink 3 times daily. For acute episodes, increase to 4 to 5 times daily.

NOTE: If taking longer than a couple of months, remove the borage every other time you make up a batch.

Makes 8 ounces

4 ounces Queen Anne's lace tincture

2 ounces burdock root tincture

1 ounce stinging nettle seed tincture

¾ ounce passionflower tincture

¼ ounce borage tincture

HEARTBREAK TEA BLEND

Heartbreak comes in many forms, from the death of a loved one to a relationship breakup. It manifests physically as chest pain and tightness, rapid heart rate and/or palpitations, and trouble breathing, or emotionally in an inability to focus, lethargy, and depression. This blend helps support the heart and relieve tension in the nervous system.

Combine all the ingredients, and store in an airtight container. Label with the list of ingredients, date, and instructions for use.

TO USE: Steep 1 tablespoon tea blend in 10 ounces of boiling water for 25 to 30 minutes. Drink 2 to 3 cups daily.

NOTE: Add a bit of honey, if desired, to sweeten.

Makes enough for 64 cups of tea

1 cup hawthorn berries
1 cup dried hawthorn leaves and flowers
1 cup dried milky oats
½ cup dried motherwort
½ cup dried reishi

INSOMNIA FORMULA

For nights when you just can't get to sleep, this formula can help, especially when you have thoughts chattering away in your mind. Take this formula right before going to bed, and keep a bottle of it at your bedside table, along with a glass of water, for a quick re-dose if needed.

1. Add the tinctures to a 1-cup glass measuring cup and stir to combine.

2. Pour the mixture into a 4-ounce glass dropper bottle.

3. Tighten the dropper lid on the bottle, then label with the list of ingredients, date, and instructions for use.

TO USE: Add 30 to 60 drops of tincture to a small glass of water or juice and drink before bed, repeating every 20 minutes if needed.

NOTE: Be sure to turn off electronic devices about an hour before bedtime to help your mind unwind. Read a book, take a relaxing bath, meditate, or do some gentle yoga exercises to get yourself in the mood for sleep.

Makes 4 ounces

1 ounce California poppy tincture

1 ounce passionflower tincture

1 ounce wild lettuce tincture

½ ounce milky oats tincture

½ ounce motherwort tincture

LACK-OF-JOY TEA TONIC

If you lack joy in your life, experiencing more downs than ups, this formula can help lift you. Motherwort and cleavers help take the edge off of things, while ginger stimulates the brain, opening your mind to receiving joy. Hawthorn supports a heavy heart, giving you courage to move into more positive emotions.

1. Add the tinctures to a 1-cup glass measuring cup and stir to combine.

2. Pour the mixture into a 4-ounce glass dropper bottle.

3. Tighten the dropper lid on the bottle, then label with the list of ingredients, date, and instructions for use.

TO USE: Add 30 to 60 drops of tincture to a small glass of water or juice and drink as needed, up to 6 times a day.

NOTE: Treat yourself to gentle exercise, such as a walk in a wooded area, a swim at your local pool, or some gentle sessions of yoga.

Makes 4 ounces

1 ounce cleavers tincture

1 ounce ginger tincture

1 ounce motherwort tincture

½ ounce hawthorn berry tincture

½ ounce hawthorn leaf and flower tincture

MENTAL STRAIN TONIC

Do you find yourself working too much? Obsessing over problems or details to the point of losing sleep? Do you push yourself to the point of not being able to "see straight"? This tonic supports and relaxes the brain and nervous system and helps improve concentration.

1. Add the tinctures to a 1-cup glass measuring cup and stir to combine.

2. Pour the mixture into a 4-ounce glass dropper bottle.

3. Tighten the dropper lid on the bottle, then label with the list of ingredients, date, and instructions for use.

TO USE: Add 40 to 60 drops of tincture to a small glass of water or juice and drink up to 4 times daily.

NOTE: Pamper yourself if you are suffering from mental strain. A long, hot bath, meditation, gentle yoga, or even a walk outdoors can help relax you and ease your mind.

Makes 4 ounces

1 ounce reishi tincture

1 ounce rosemary tincture

½ ounce gotu kola tincture

½ ounce milky oats tincture

½ ounce motherwort tincture

½ ounce passionflower tincture

POST-TRAUMATIC STRESS DISORDER FORMULA

PTSD can strike at any time after you experience something extremely shocking, frightening, or dangerous. This formula helps calm the reactive state of the brain, lessening the length and frequency of episodes and helping you stay calm during an episode as you work through the trauma.

1. Add the tinctures to a 1-cup glass measuring cup and stir to combine.

2. Pour the mixture into an 8-ounce glass dropper bottle.

3. Tighten the dropper lid on the bottle, then label with the list of ingredients, date, and instructions for use.

Makes 8 ounces

4 ounces borage tincture

2 ounces gotu kola tincture

2 ounces wild lettuce tincture

TO USE: Add 10 to 30 drops of tincture to a small glass of water or juice and drink 3 times daily. For acute episodes, increase to 4 to 5 times daily. If taking long term, take a 1 week break after every 4 weeks of taking the formula.

NOTE: Be sure to support yourself with plenty of rest, exercise, water, and a wholesome diet.

STRESS RELIEF TEA BLEND

If you are feeling stressed, supporting your nervous system with a cup of this tea can help you relax. The combination of herbs nourishes and strengthens the nervous system and supports the liver to help your body process stress in a healthier way. The flavor is rich and earthy with a hint of sweetness. Adding a bit of honey and cream makes it a perfect drink to unwind with after a long day.

Combine all the ingredients, and store in an airtight container. Label with the list of ingredients, date, and instructions for use.

TO USE: Steep 2 teaspoons of the tea blend in 8 ounces of boiling water for 20 to 30 minutes. Drink 2 to 3 cups daily.

NOTE: Add honey to sweeten, if desired.

Makes enough for 60 cups of tea

1 cup dried burdock root

1 cup dried milky oats

½ cup dried
   California poppy

VITALITY-BOOSTING TEA BLEND

Vitality comes from the Latin word vita, *which means "life." Having low vitality means not living your life to the fullest. If you are feeling low or uninspired, try a cup of this vitality-boosting tea to help increase your zest for life. The herbs in this blend will nourish and support your energy flow.*

Combine all the ingredients, and store in an air-tight container. Label with the list of ingredients, date, and instructions for use.

TO USE: Steep 2 teaspoons of the tea blend in 8 ounces of boiling water for 15 to 20 minutes. Drink 2 to 3 cups daily.

NOTE: Sweeten with a bit of honey, if desired.

Makes enough for 60 cups of tea

1 cup dried lemon balm

1 cup dried stinging nettle leaves

½ cup dried burdock root

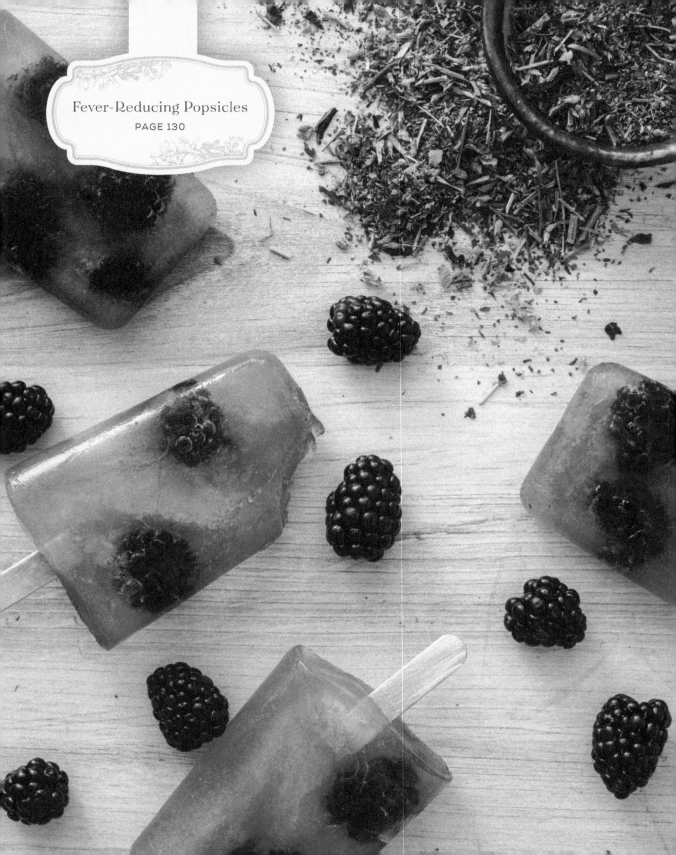

Fever-Reducing Popsicles
PAGE 130

CHAPTER SIX

COMMON CHILDHOOD CONDITIONS

Kids come with their own varieties of ailments, and most of these recipes are focused on childhood ailments that pop up around the teen years. (See the Resources section on page 227 for information about where to find recipes for babies.) From chickenpox, conjunctivitis, pertussis, and strep throat, to sore throats, stomachaches, warts, and lice, this chapter has your kids covered. Even when it comes to fevers, earaches, and worms, help can be found in your herbal pantry.

Teens in particular will experience relief with the Hormonal Mood Swing Formula (page 131), Acne Formula (page 123), and Deep Cystic Acne Formula (page 128) recipes. All of these recipes are easy to follow and go over well with kids, given their mild flavors and gentle herbs.

ACNE FORMULA

This formula supports the liver and helps clear acne. Burdock and wild lettuce may be slow to act, but they work deeply for lasting effects. Gotu kola repairs damaged skin, while vitex balances hormones.

1. Add the tinctures to a 1-cup glass measuring cup and stir to combine.

2. Pour the mixture into an 8-ounce glass dropper bottle.

3. Tighten the dropper lid on the bottle, then label with the list of ingredients, date, and instructions for use.

Makes 8 ounces

4 ounces burdock root tincture
2 ounces gotu kola tincture
1½ ounces vitex tincture
½ ounce wild lettuce tincture

TO USE: Add 30 drops of tincture to a small glass of water or juice and drink 3 times daily for at least 3 months.

NOTE: Avoid excessive amounts of sugar, caffeine, and processed foods that bog down the liver and impair its functioning.

ADD/ADHD ELIXIR

Symptoms of Attention-Deficit Disorder (ADD) and Attention-Deficit/Hyperactivity Disorder (ADHD) include impulsive behaviors, difficulty paying attention, and fidgeting, among other behaviors. The herbs in this formula calm the mind, improve focus and concentration, and reduce agitation.

1. Combine the tinctures and honey into a 1-cup glass measuring cup and stir to combine. If the honey is thick, gently heat it first to make it pourable.

2. Pour the elixir into an 8-ounce glass dropper bottle.

3. Tighten the dropper lid on the bottle, then label with the list of ingredients, date, and instructions for use.

TO USE: Take 10 to 30 drops 3 times daily.

NOTE: Diet often plays a huge role in children's behaviors. While this herbal elixir can go a long way to improve the symptoms of ADD/ADHD, consult a health care practitioner and review foods that may be contributing to their difficulties, such as wheat, corn, dairy, preservatives, or artificial colors and flavorings, to find ways to increase your child's quality of life.

Makes 8 ounces

1 ounce California poppy tincture

1 ounce catnip tincture

1 ounce gotu kola tincture

1 ounce passionflower tincture

1 ounce St. John's wort tincture

½ ounce hawthorn berry tincture

½ ounce wild lettuce tincture

1 ounce honey

BEDWETTING RELIEF ELIXIR

Bedwetting can be caused by many things, from an immature bladder to deep sleep or a lack of hormones that decrease the production of urine. It often goes away on its own with time. If bedwetting is a common occurrence in your household, this elixir may help bring about relief by supporting the bladder and helping suppress the urge to urinate.

1. Combine the tinctures and honey into a 1-cup glass measuring cup and stir to combine. If the honey is thick, gently heat first to thin.

2. Pour the elixir into a 2-ounce glass dropper bottle.

3. Tighten the dropper lid on the bottle, then label with the list of ingredients, date, and instructions for use.

Makes 2 ounces

1 ounce St. John's wort tincture

½ ounce California poppy tincture

½ ounce honey

TO USE: Take 20 to 30 drops 1 to 2 hours before bed. Can be repeated with a second dose at bedtime.

NOTE: If bedwetting becomes chronic, consult a health care practitioner to rule out a medical condition such as a bladder infection.

BULLY-BE-GONE TEA BLEND

If your child is being bullied, this tea can help ease their nervous tension as the situation is being resolved. On the flip side, these herbs also can be used to help calm a child who is acting like a bully and encourage them to work through their behavior.

Combine all the ingredients, and store in an airtight container. Label with the list of ingredients, date, and instructions for use.

Makes enough for 48 cups of tea

½ cup dried catnip

½ cup hawthorn berries

½ cup dried milky oats

¼ cup dried borage flowers

¼ cup dried wild cherry

TO USE: Steep 2 teaspoons of the tea blend in 8 ounces of boiling water for 15 to 20 minutes. Drink 1 to 2 cups daily.

NOTE: Sweeten with a bit of honey, if desired.

CHICKENPOX ELIXIR

Chickenpox can make a child feel miserable. This formula supports and soothes the nervous system, reduce fevers and itchiness, and promotes quick healing.

1. Combine the tinctures and honey into a 1-cup glass measuring cup and stir to combine. If the honey is thick, gently heat first to thin.

2. Use a small metal funnel to pour the tincture into a 4-ounce glass dropper bottle.

3. Tighten the dropper lid on the bottle, then label with the list of ingredients, date, and instructions for use.

Makes 4 ounces

1 ounce lemon balm tincture

½ ounce black walnut leaf tincture

½ ounce milky oats tincture

½ ounce yarrow tincture

½ ounce prunella tincture

½ ounce spilanthes tincture

½ ounce honey

TO USE: Take 10 to 30 drops 4 to 6 times daily.

NOTE: For extra healing and relief, use oatmeal baths, and apply chamomile essential oil to rashes.

CONJUNCTIVITIS AND STYE EYE WASH

Sometimes referred to as "pinkeye," conjunctivitis is an inflammation of the clear tissue that surrounds the white of the eye and the insides of the eyelid. The white of the eye turns pink, and there can be itching, pain, burning, or a scratchy feeling caused by an allergy, bacteria, or a virus. Soothe irritated eyes with this eye wash blend, which contains a variety of herbs that have antiviral and antihistamine properties. If you suspect a bacterial infection, you can use this along with an oral antibiotic.

Combine all the herbs in an airtight container. Label with the list of ingredients, date, and instructions for use.

TO USE: Steep 2 teaspoons of the tea blend in 8 ounces of boiling water for 15 to 20 minutes, adding 1 teaspoon sea salt to the blend and stirring to dissolve. When the tea has cooled, strain it through a fine-mesh sieve into a clean eye cup. Ask your child to lean forward, and place the cup tightly against their eye. Next, have them open their eye and stand upright, flipping their head back so their face is looking at the ceiling. Have your child blink several times and then bend forward again. Repeat these steps with fresh tea on the other eye, if needed. Rinse the eyes 4 to 5 times daily until they are completely clear of any irritation.

NOTE: The tea can be brewed, strained, and refrigerated for 3 to 4 days.

Makes 4 cups

2 teaspoons dried thyme

2 teaspoons dried ground ivy

2 teaspoons dried gotu kola

1 teaspoon dried goldenrod

1 teaspoon dried prunella

1 teaspoon sea salt (per dose)

DEEP CYSTIC ACNE FORMULA

When using this formula, cystic acne will gradually decrease until it's cleared up, but it's not uncommon for the acne to reappear. Continue with another regimen of this formula if you experience a flare-up, and the second round should clear up as well. This herbal remedy may be slow-acting, but the results are worth the wait.

1. Add the tinctures to a 1-cup glass measuring cup and stir to combine.

2. Pour the mixture into an 8-ounce glass dropper bottle.

3. Tighten the dropper lid on the bottle, then label with the list of ingredients, date, and instructions for use.

TO USE: Add 30 drops of tincture to a small glass of water or juice and drink 3 times daily.

NOTE: This formula can take a few months to work. For a better outcome, be sure your teen is getting plenty of water and wholesome foods in their diet, along with some daily exercise.

Makes 8 ounces

2 ounces burdock root tincture

2 ounces saw palmetto tincture

2 ounces vitex tincture

2 ounces wild lettuce tincture

EARACHE OIL

Few things make a child more miserable than an earache. After applying this oil, cover the ear with a hot water bottle or warmed sock filled with salt for extra soothing relief. St. John's wort and plantain both ease earache pain and fight infection.

1. Combine the oils together in a glass measuring cup and stir to combine.

2. Pour into a 1-ounce bottle.

3. Tighten the lid on the bottle, then label with the list of ingredients, date, and instructions for use. Store in the refrigerator, and discard at the first sign of rancidity.

TO USE: Have your child lay on their side with the painful ear facing up. Put 5 to 10 drops of oil into the ear and plug it with a cotton ball. After 5 to 10 minutes, repeat the process in the other ear. Repeat every 2 to 4 hours as needed.

NOTE: Do not use this oil if you suspect a ruptured eardrum.

Makes 1 ounce

½ ounce St. John's wort–infused oil
½ ounce plantain-infused oil

FEVER-REDUCING POPSICLES

Fevers are the body's natural response to killing germs in our body, and we generally should support them and allow them to do their job. If your child is extremely uncomfortable or the fever is climbing beyond your comfort level, try these popsicles that contain herbs to lower it without medications that can tax the liver. This blend of herbs helps lower fever and ease accompanying body aches—and it tastes delicious.

Combine all the ingredients (except for black-berries), and store in an airtight container. Label with the list of ingredients, date, and instructions for use.

TO USE: Steep ¼ cup of the tea blend in 1 quart of boiling water for 15 to 20 minutes. Cool and pour into Popsicle molds for easy freezing. If using blackberries, put 3 to 5 in each mold before adding the tea. You may wish to add a tablespoon of honey if your child prefers them sweeter.

NOTE: This recipe can be used as a tea, too, if your child is cold and prefers not to have Popsicles. It also can be brewed as a bath tea to help reduce fever. Instructions for making an herbal bath can be found on page 73.

Makes 128 (2-ounce) Popsicles or 32 cups of tea

½ cup dried spearmint

½ cup dried prunella

¼ cup dried monarda

¼ cup dried catnip

¼ cup dried blackberry leaves

2 tablespoons dried yarrow

2 tablespoons dried goldenrod

Fresh or frozen blackberries (optional)

HORMONAL MOOD SWING FORMULA

The teen years can be rocky as hormones fluctuate. Herbal support can bring about a natural balance, helping teens feel more confident, less irrational, and in a better mood. The herbs in this formula support the liver and calm the endocrine system during this tumultuous period of life.

1. Add the tinctures to a 1-cup glass measuring cup and stir to combine.

2. Pour the mixture into a 4-ounce glass dropper bottle.

3. Tighten the dropper lid on the bottle, then label with the list of ingredients, date, and instructions for use.

Makes 4 ounces

1 ounce burdock root tincture

1 ounce stinging nettle leaf tincture

1 ounce vitex tincture

1 ounce motherwort tincture

TO USE: Add 30 to 40 drops of tincture to a small glass of water or juice, and drink 3 times daily for a minimum of 3 months. Once hormones have remained in balance for at least a month, reduce the dose to twice daily for another month, then to once daily for a final month.

NOTE: Teens need to be drinking plenty of water (about half their weight in ounces is a good starting point), and they also need to eat a wholesome diet with minimal processed foods and sugar, exercise, and get 8 to 10 hours of sleep daily.

IMMUNE SYSTEM BOOST & SUPPORT TONIC ELIXIR

This elixir can be used as a daily tonic to support and tone the immune system. It also can be taken in increased doses at the first sign of symptoms to prevent an illness or lessen its duration.

1. Combine the tinctures and honey in a 1-cup glass measuring cup and stir to combine. If the honey is thick, gently heat first to thin.

2. Pour the elixir into an 8-ounce glass dropper bottle.

3. Tighten the dropper lid on the bottle, then label with the list of ingredients, date, and instructions for use.

Makes 8 ounces

2 ounces spilanthes tincture

1 ounce blackberry leaf tincture

1 ounce gotu kola tincture

1 ounce monarda tincture

1 ounce prunella tincture

1 ounce reishi tincture

1 ounce honey

TO USE: Take 10 to 30 drops 3 times daily. For acute episodes, increase to 4 to 5 times daily.

NOTE: Consider a daily vitamin D_3 supplement (up to 2,000 IUs per day) to help boost the immune system.

LARYNGITIS RELIEF HONEY

Honey coats the throat and soothes inflammation, and the herbs in this recipe fight infection and ease irritations to help heal the throat. The sweetness of the honey balances perfectly with the pungency of the herbs, making this a sweet tasting remedy.

1. Combine the herbs and honey in a small saucepan, stirring well.

2. Cover and let the mixture steep for at least 2 hours. Place the pan over low heat and warm the honey just until it is liquefied and pourable.

3. Line a fine-mesh sieve with a thin, clean cloth and strain the honey into a clean jar.

4. Let the honey cool to room temperature, then seal the jar and label it with the list of ingredients, date, and instructions for use.

Makes 6 to 18 doses

1 teaspoon dried
  calendula flower petals
1 teaspoon dried prunella
1 teaspoon dried thyme
¼ teaspoon dried black
  walnut leaves
1 fresh poke berry (with the
  seed removed)
¼ cup honey

TO USE: Swallow 1 to 3 teaspoons every 30 minutes for the first hour, then take 1 to 3 teaspoons every 2 to 3 hours as needed.

NOTE: This honey also can be added to a tea of thyme, prunella, or rosemary that you can drink hot 2 to 3 times over the course of a day. To make the tea, steep 1 to 3 teaspoons of any of the herbs in this recipe in 8 ounces of boiling water for 15 minutes. Add 1 to 3 teaspoons of honey.

LICE-BE-GONE OIL

Lice means misery for any household. This formula suffocates lice to eliminate them without the use of harsh and potentially toxic chemicals such as permethrin. Because this oil contains natural, infused plants, the lice do not develop resistance to it as they do to many over-the-counter medications.

1. Combine the oils together in a glass measuring cup and stir to combine.

2. Pour into a 4-ounce bottle.

3. Tighten the lid on the bottle, and label with the list of ingredients, date, and instructions for use. Store in the refrigerator, and discard at the first sign of rancidity.

Makes 4 ounces

2 ounces black walnut leaf–infused oil

1 ounce rosemary-infused oil

1 ounce thyme-infused oil

TO USE: Apply a liberal amount of oil to the scalp and massage. Cover with a shower cap and leave on for 30 minutes before running a lice comb through the scalp. Rinse with warm water followed by shampoo. Repeat as needed.

NOTE: Don't share a comb or hairbrush if someone in your household has lice. Be sure to wash bedding, hats, etc. in hot water to kill off any remaining lice.

MOTION SICKNESS LOZENGES

If your child suffers from motion sickness, they can dread long car rides. These lozenges are handy to have on hand; they taste sweet and spicy, with a hint of mint, and they help soothe upset stomachs.

1. Follow the instructions on page 69 to make a syrup (using all the ingredients except for the powdered sugar), and continue to heat and simmer syrup until it reaches hard ball stage (around 260°F on a candy thermometer).

2. While the syrup heats, line a rimmed baking sheet with parchment paper. Grease the parchment paper with butter.

3. Once the syrup reaches the hard ball stage, pour it onto the parchment paper and let it cool.

4. When the syrup is halfway cool, use a knife to score it into nickel-size pieces.

5. When the syrup is completely cooled, break it along the score lines. Toss the pieces with powdered sugar.

6. Store the lozenges in an airtight container. Label with the list of ingredients, date, and instructions for use.

Makes 36 to 48 drops

¼ cup dried ginger

2 tablespoons dried spearmint

1 tablespoon dried catnip

16 ounces water

8 ounces honey

powdered sugar (for coating)

TO USE: Suck on 1 lozenge as needed.

NOTE: This recipe can be used as a syrup if you prefer not to make lozenges.

NIGHT TERRORS AND NIGHTMARES FORMULA

Children have night terrors generally around 1½ hours after they fall asleep, and they usually don't remember them the next day. Nightmares, on the other hand, tend to happen during the middle of night or early morning when children are in a lighter stage of sleep, and they can usually be remembered. These two herbs are my favorite for helping ease both night terrors and nightmares: Mugwort helps to ease night terrors, and catnip supports the nervous system and helps relax the mind.

1. Add the tinctures to a 1-cup glass measuring cup and stir to combine.

2. Pour the mixture into a 2-ounce glass dropper bottle.

3. Tighten the dropper lid on the bottle, then label with the list of ingredients, date, and instructions for use.

Makes 2 ounces

1 ounce mugwort tincture
1 ounce catnip tincture

TO USE: Add 10 to 30 drops of tincture to a small glass of water or juice and drink before bed. If needed, take 2 doses—the first 1 hour before bed and the second at bedtime.

NOTE: Children are very sensitive to the healing power of stones and crystals. Try giving your child a piece of rose quartz or selenite to put under their pillow for extra security at night.

NOSEBLEED POWDER

This powder is great for stopping nosebleeds and other bleeding as well.

Combine the powders together and stir until well mixed. Store in an airtight bottle. Label with the list of ingredients, date, and instructions for use.

TO USE: Sprinkle on an open wound. Can be used as a snuff in the nose for nosebleeds, or a couple pinches can be placed in the nose to help stop the bleeding. Use as needed.

NOTE: I learned from herbalist Susan Marynowski to use an empty Tic-Tac container as a small travel-size powder dispenser. It works great to shake out a little powder as needed.

Makes 2 tablespoons

1 tablespoon powdered dried yarrow

1 tablespoon powdered dried plantain

PERTUSSIS TEA BLEND

Pertussis, commonly known as whooping cough, is a highly contagious respiratory disease. It gets its name from the characteristic "whoop" sound of the cough. This tea blend helps to relax the bronchial tubes to help lessen the spasmodic coughing of pertussis and other respiratory ailments. It also helps to expectorate mucus and debris from the lungs and bronchial passages.

Combine all the ingredients, and store in an airtight container. Label with the list of ingredients, date, and instructions for use.

TO USE: Steep 2 teaspoons of the tea blend in 8 ounces of boiling water for 15 to 20 minutes. Drink ½ to 1 cup as needed. Sweeten with a bit of honey, if desired.

NOTE: This blend also can be made into an elixir for late-night dosing when spasmodic coughs seem to be more problematic.

Makes enough for 48 cups of tea

½ cup dried wild cherry

½ cup dried New England aster

¼ cup dried goldenrod

¼ cup dried monarda

¼ cup dried thyme

¼ cup dried wild lettuce

SORE THROAT GARGLE

Sore throats can be soothed with this blend of herbs, which also helps kill off viruses. These herbs help combat germs, reduce inflammation, and relieve pain.

Combine all the ingredients except the salt in an airtight container. Label with the list of ingredients, date, and instructions for use.

TO USE: Steep 2 teaspoons of the tea blend in 8 ounces of boiling water for 15 to 20 minutes, then add 2 to 3 teaspoons of sea salt and stir to dissolve. Allow to cool enough to gargle. Repeat as needed for relief.

NOTE: If your child doesn't like gargling, omit the sea salt and use this as a tea blend sweetened with a bit of honey. Have them drink 1 to 2 cups throughout the day.

Makes enough for 24 gargle cups

¼ cup dried
   blackberry leaves
¼ cup dried ginger
¼ cup dried ground ivy
¼ cup dried prunella
2 to 3 teaspoons sea salt

STOMACHACHE TEA BLEND

Help soothe digestive troubles and tummy aches with this digestive tea blend. This tea works well for all types of stomachaches and can help relieve gas and bloating, too.

Combine all the ingredients, and store in an airtight container. Label with the list of ingredients, date, and instructions for use.

Makes enough for 48 cups of tea

1 cup dried dandelion root
½ cup dried ginger
½ cup dried thyme

TO USE: Steep 2 teaspoons of the tea blend in 8 ounces of boiling water for 20 to 25 minutes. Drink ½ to 1 cup as needed.

NOTE: Sweeten with a bit of honey, if desired.

WART REDUCER OIL

Warts are skin growths caused by the human papilloma virus that typically appear on the hands, feet, or genitals. Ginger and calendula are antiviral and help kill off warts.

1. Combine the oils in a glass measuring cup and stir to combine.

2. Pour into a 2-ounce bottle.

3. Tighten the lid on the bottle, then label with the list of ingredients, date, and instructions for use. Store in the refrigerator, and discard at the first sign of rancidity.

Makes 2 ounces

1 ounce ginger-infused oil
1 ounce calendula-
   infused oil

TO USE: Massage into the warts, then apply a Band-Aid. Reapply twice daily until warts are gone.

NOTE: Securing the Band-Aid with duct tape or surgical tape can hasten healing.

WATER-IN-THE-EAR DROPS

Water in the ear is a common problem for people who spend a lot of time swimming or participating in water-based activities such as surfing. When water stays in the ear canal, it can lead to inflammation and infection. Yarrow helps to draw out water from the ear and prevent infection while reducing inflammation.

Pour into a 1-ounce bottle. Label the bottle with the formula name, ingredients, and instructions for use.

Makes 1 ounce

1 ounce yarrow tincture

TO USE: Have your child lay on their side. Add 5 to 10 drops of tincture into the ear, and gently massage around the base of the ear. After 5 to 10 minutes, repeat the process in the other ear. If needed, follow up with some Earache Oil (page 129).

NOTE: Use this after your child has been swimming as a preventative measure.

WORM FORMULA

This blend of herbs helps to stun, kill, and expel worms such as pinworms, thread worms, and tapeworms from the digestive tract.

1. Add the tinctures to a 1-cup glass measuring cup, and stir to combine.

2. Pour the mixture into a 2-ounce glass dropper bottle.

3. Tighten the dropper lid on the bottle, then label with the list of ingredients, date, and instructions for use.

Makes 2 ounces

½ ounce black walnut tincture
½ ounce thyme tincture
½ ounce mugwort tincture
½ ounce ginger tincture

TO USE: Take 10 to 30 drops 3 times daily for 14 days. Repeat if needed.

NOTE: Just a bit of honey can sweeten the formula so kids can tolerate the bitter herbs that expel worms. Add about ⅛ to ¼ ounce honey to the mix if needed.

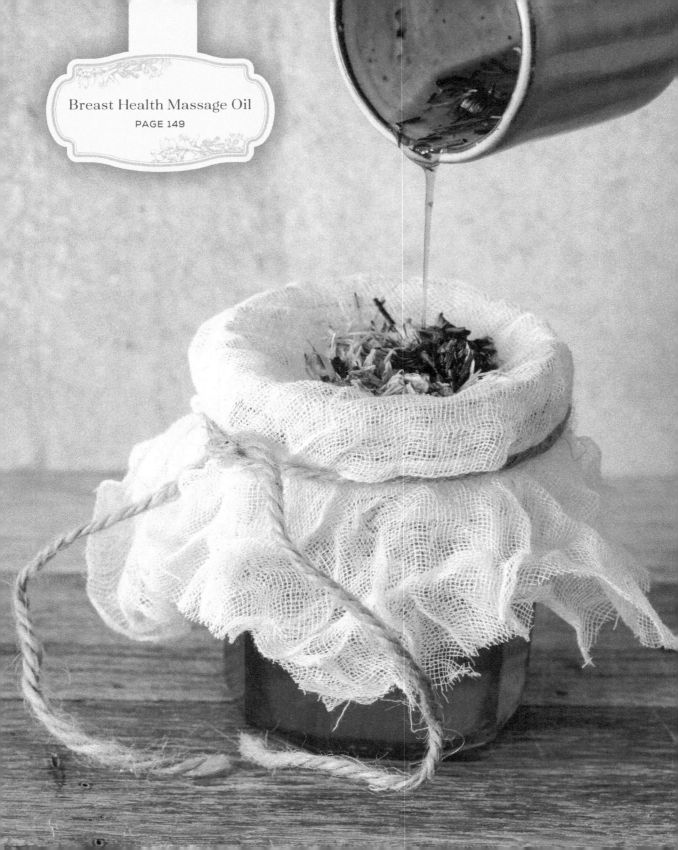

Breast Health Massage Oil
PAGE 149

CHAPTER SEVEN

WOMEN'S HEALTH

As women, we are often busy, putting the needs of our jobs and family before ourselves. In this chapter, you'll find remedies for everything from fatigue (see Adrenal Health Tonic [page 147] and Endocrine System Support Formula [page 152]) to anemia (see Iron-Building Tonic Syrup [page 154]).

You'll also find herbal medicines to relieve other common female ailments such as bladder infections and yeast infections, as well as PMS and menstrual cramps, without the side effects of pharmaceuticals. And if you're experiencing perimenopause or menopause, I've got you covered with recipes that address hot flashes and night sweats, breast health, weight loss, and calcium building support.

There's a long history of women using remedies with herbs that are powerful and effective. Start discovering just how easy it can be to find herb-based health relief and support.

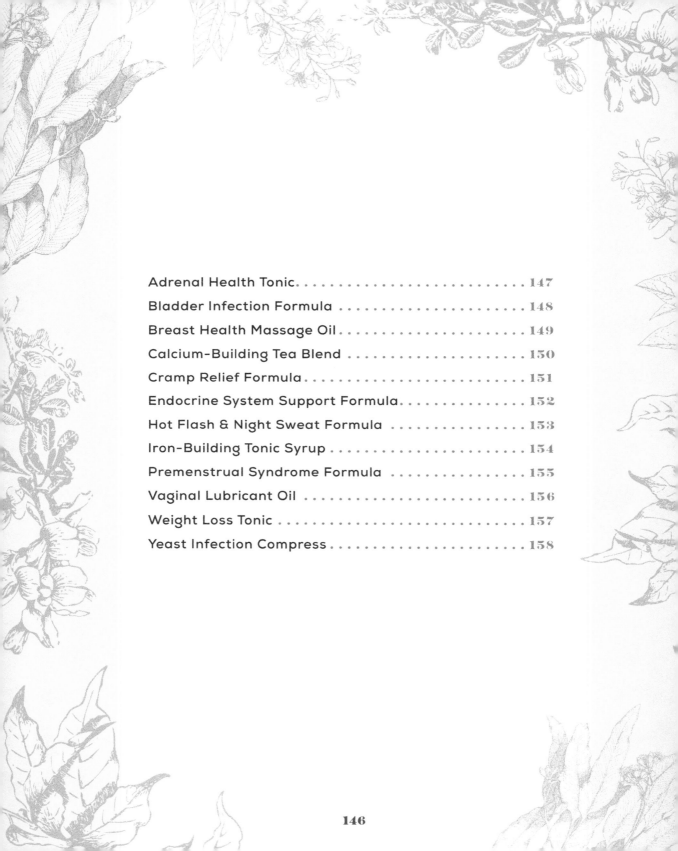

ADRENAL HEALTH TONIC

Adrenal fatigue, also known as adrenal insufficiency, refers to the body's inability to produce enough hormones due to some underlying issue or disease. The symptoms include body aches, weight loss without any dietary or lifestyle changes, fatigue, low blood pressure, thinning body hair, skin pigmentation, insomnia, digestive issues, and nervousness. This tonic rebuilds the adrenals while relaxing the nervous system.

1. Add the tinctures to a 1-cup glass measuring cup and stir to combine.

2. Pour the mixture into an 8-ounce glass dropper bottle.

3. Tighten the dropper lid on the bottle, then label with the list of ingredients, date, and instructions for use.

Makes 8 ounces

3 ounces Queen Anne's lace tincture

3 ounces stinging nettle tincture

2 ounces milky oats tincture

TO USE: Add 30 to 40 drops of tincture to a small glass of water or juice and drink 3 times daily for at least 3 months.

NOTE: While this tonic can help support and nourish the adrenals, it's important to take additional steps to truly heal and replenish your adrenal system. Combine this tonic with other supportive health measures, including saying no when you need to, getting enough rest, and doing meditation and/or yoga.

BLADDER INFECTION FORMULA

Bladder infections tend to appear out of the blue, presenting with painful urination and blood in the urine. They can affect all parts of the urinary tract, including the bladder, kidneys, ureters, and the urethra. This formula has antibacterial and diuretic properties, helping to remove all traces of bacteria, relieving pain, and changing the pH of urine to make it harder for bacteria to grow in the bladder.

1. Add the tinctures to a 1-cup glass measuring cup and stir to combine.

2. Pour the mixture into an 8-ounce glass dropper bottle.

3. Tighten the dropper lid on the bottle, then label with the list of ingredients, date, and instructions for use.

TO USE: Add 30 to 40 drops of tincture to a small glass of water or juice, and drink 4 to 6 times daily. Continue taking for 3 days after all signs of infection are gone.

NOTE: Drink lots of water and unsweetened cranberry juice to increase the formula's effectiveness.

Makes 8 ounces

2 ounces Queen Anne's lace tincture

2 ounces spilanthes tincture

1½ ounces goldenrod tincture

1 ounce ground ivy tincture

½ ounce cleavers tincture

½ ounce monarda tincture

½ ounce yarrow tincture

BREAST HEALTH MASSAGE OIL

As we age, our breasts can develop lumps that appear during or around ovulation and disappear at the start of menses. While these lumps are perfectly normal, they can be tender to the touch. This oil helps to maintain breast health while breaking down cysts in the breast.

1. Add the oils to a glass measuring cup and stir to combine.

2. Pour into a 4-ounce bottle.

3. Tighten the lid on the bottle, then label with the list of ingredients, date, and instructions for use. Store in the refrigerator, and discard at the first sign of rancidity.

TO USE: Massage into breasts as needed. For cysts, massage 2 to 3 times daily. If nursing, be sure to wipe off all oil before letting the baby latch on.

NOTE: Monthly breast self-exams are important for noting any changes to breast tissue. Consult your health care practitioner if you have concerns about a cyst that does not go away or if you notice anything suspicious.

Makes 4 ounces

2 ounces calendula-infused oil

1½ ounces cleavers-infused oil

½ ounce poke root–infused oil

CALCIUM-BUILDING TEA BLEND

Our bodies store calcium in the bones and teeth, but we need this nutrient throughout our body for muscle and nerve function, vascular dilation and contraction, hormonal secretion, and more. As we age, our bodies are slowly depleted of calcium, which is leached from our bones and teeth, weakening them. This tea blend helps return calcium to the bones.

Combine all the ingredients, and store in an airtight container. Label with the list of ingredients, date, and instructions for use.

TO USE: Steep 1 tablespoon tea blend in 8 ounces of boiling water for 25 to 30 minutes. Drink 2 to 3 cups daily. Add a bit of honey to sweeten, if desired.

NOTE: Calcium works best in conjunction with magnesium, so consider taking a daily magnesium citrate supplement in the evening before bed.

Makes enough for 64 cups of tea

1½ cups dried milky oats
1 cup dried stinging
   nettle leaves
½ cup dried
   blackberry leaves
½ cup dried lemon balm
½ cup dried burdock root

CRAMP RELIEF FORMULA

Menstrual cramps can be a normal part of a women's menstrual cycle or an indication of an underlying condition such as endometriosis or uterine fibroids. For general menstrual cramping, this formula is antispasmodic and works fast to provide relief. It also can be used for other muscle cramps.

1. Add the tinctures to a 1-cup glass measuring cup and stir to combine.

2. Pour the mixture into a 4-ounce glass dropper bottle.

3. Tighten the dropper lid on the bottle, then label with the list of ingredients, date, and instructions for use.

Makes 4 ounces

2 ounces motherwort tincture

2 ounces black haw tincture

TO USE: Add 30 to 40 drops of tincture to a small glass of water or juice, and drink 3 times daily. Dosage can be increased to every 20 minutes for 1 to 2 hours to relieve cramping, if needed.

NOTE: Take it easy on yourself when you have menstrual cramps. Lying down with a hot water bottle on your stomach can be calming, helping to relax you as the herbs kick in.

ENDOCRINE SYSTEM SUPPORT FORMULA

Feeling run down with your hormones all over the place? This formula helps to balance the endocrine system while calming the nervous system. Queen Anne's lace and vitex are not the best tasting herbs, so using these herbs in a formula instead of a tea makes them easier to take on a regular basis.

1. Add the tinctures to a 1-cup glass measuring cup and stir to combine.

2. Pour the mixture into an 8-ounce glass dropper bottle.

3. Tighten the dropper lid on the bottle, then label with the list of ingredients, date, and instructions for use.

Makes 4 ounces

1½ ounces Queen Anne's lace tincture
1½ ounces vitex tincture
1 ounce milky oats tincture

TO USE: Add 30 to 40 drops of tincture to a small glass of water or juice, and drink 3 times daily.

NOTE: Stress and sleep deprivation are two big culprits behind adrenal insufficiency. Be sure to get plenty of rest, and learn to practice stress-reducing activities such as meditation, yoga, walking, or another gentle exercise.

HOT FLASH & NIGHT SWEAT FORMULA

This formula balances hormones while providing relief from hot flashes and night sweats. It also calms heart palpitations and stabilizes progesterone so hot flashes and night sweats become a thing of the past and you can remain comfortable day and night during menopause.

1. Add the tinctures to a 1-cup glass measuring cup and stir to combine.

2. Pour the mixture into an 8-ounce glass dropper bottle.

3. Tighten the dropper lid on the bottle, then label with the list of ingredients, date, and instructions for use.

TO USE: Add 40 to 60 drops of tincture to a small glass of water or juice, and drink 4 to 6 times daily. After 2 weeks, cut back to 30 to 40 drops 4 to 6 times daily. After another 2 weeks, cut back to 30 to 40 drops 3 times daily. Continue cutting back, increasing the dosage only if hot flashes and night sweats recur.

NOTE: If your menopause symptoms are severely uncomfortable and you aren't getting enough relief with this formula, consider seeing an acupuncturist to alleviate your symptoms. While herbs can go a long way, sometimes they work best with other alternative therapies.

Makes 8 ounces

2 ounces borage flower tincture

2 ounces motherwort tincture

2 ounces vitex tincture

1 ounce blackberry leaf tincture

1 ounce yarrow tincture

IRON-BUILDING TONIC SYRUP

Women often experience iron deficiency due to menstruation, which removes blood and iron from our system every month. This formula, a variation on a recipe I learned from herbalist Rosemary Gladstar, helps the body absorb and process iron more efficiently. The flavor tastes strongly of molasses and cherries, almost like a dessert cordial.

1. Follow the instructions on page 69 to make a syrup, using the blackstrap molasses instead of honey.

2. Label with the list of ingredients, date, and instructions for use. Store in the refrigerator. Use within 3 months.

TO USE: Take 4 to 6 tablespoons daily.

NOTE: This is an effective tonic that can be taken on a long-term basis. I know many women who take this formula or a similar one as part of their daily regimen for months or years. Some find they only need to take it for 2 weeks each month after their menses begin.

Makes 16 ounces

1½ cups dried
blackberry root

1½ cups dried
dandelion root

1½ cups dried
dandelion leaves

1½ cups dried stinging
nettle leaves

½ cup dried yellow
dock root

½ cup dried burdock root

½ cup hawthorn berries

½ cup dried lemon balm

4 ounces blackstrap
molasses

¼ cup brandy

¼ cup black cherry fruit
concentrate (not juice)

PREMENSTRUAL SYNDROME FORMULA

Premenstrual syndrome (PMS) can present in a variety of ways, including acne, tender breasts, mood swings, food cravings, bloating, tiredness, and irritability. This formula helps to reduce the symptoms of PMS by balancing hormones. For best results, take it throughout the month.

1. Add the tinctures to a 1-cup glass measuring cup and stir to combine.

2. Pour the mixture into an 8-ounce glass dropper bottle.

3. Tighten the dropper lid on the bottle, then label with the list of ingredients, date, and instructions for use.

Makes 8 ounces

2 ounces motherwort tincture

2 ounces vitex tincture

2 ounces lemon balm tincture

1 ounce cleavers tincture

1 ounce milky oats tincture

TO USE: Add 20 to 40 drops of the formula to a small glass of water or juice, and drink 3 times daily. For acute episodes, increase to 4 to 5 times daily.

NOTE: Regular exercise, a wholesome diet, and plenty of rest also can help reduce the symptoms of PMS.

VAGINAL LUBRICANT OIL

As women age and head into menopause, we lose our natural ability to lubricate, and intimacy can become uncomfortable. The herbs in this oil help lubricate the vagina to make sex pleasurable again.

Makes 4 ounces

2 ounces gotu kola–infused oil

2 ounces milky oat–infused oil

1. Combine the oils together in a glass measuring cup and stir to combine.

2. Pour into a 4-ounce bottle.

3. Tighten the lid on the bottle, then label with the list of ingredients, date, and instructions for use.

4. Store in the refrigerator, and discard at the first sign of rancidity.

TO USE: Apply twice daily and immediately before getting intimate.

NOTE: Drink milky oat infusions (pages 26 to 27) several times a week to improve vaginal hydration levels.

WEIGHT LOSS TONIC

The best way to lose weight is to eat wholesome, nutrient-rich foods and get lots of exercise. However, this formula can play a supporting role in your weight loss initiative by improving digestion and circulation and supporting the endocrine system. The water dilutes any strong flavors from the tinctures.

1. Add the tinctures to a 1-cup glass measuring cup and stir to combine.

2. Use a small metal funnel to pour the tincture into an 8-ounce glass dropper bottle.

3. Tighten the dropper lid on the bottle, then label with the list of ingredients, date, and instructions for use.

TO USE: Add 30 to 40 drops of tincture to a small glass of water or juice, and drink 3 times daily.

NOTE: Look for fun dance routine exercises to help remove stubborn fat—they help get the lymph flowing, really work the core muscles, and are just plain fun! If you're not into dance, try another invigorating exercise routine that works your core muscles and gets you moving to increase the formula's effectiveness.

Makes 8 ounces

4 ounces Queen Anne's lace tincture

2 ounces reishi tincture

1 ounce ginger tincture

1 ounce dandelion leaf tincture

YEAST INFECTION COMPRESS

This formula works well for all types of yeast infections caused by an over-growth of the fungi Candida albicans. The biggest symptom is intense burning and itching in the vagina or on the nipples, the latter of which is known as thrush and is common among breastfeeding women. If you are suffering from thrush, be sure to apply the compress to your baby, too. Take a cloth dipped in this compress and wipe it around the inside of baby's mouth before and after nursing.

Makes enough for 6 quarts of tea for compresses

1 cup dried black
   walnut leaves
1 cup dried burdock leaves
½ cup dried monarda
¼ cup dried plantain
¼ cup dried yellow
   dock root

1. Combine the herbs in a bowl and stir to blend. Store in a half gallon jar. Label with the list of ingredients, date, and instructions for use.

2. To make your compress, boil 1 quart of water.

3. Add ½ cup of the herbal blend to a quart jar and pour in enough boiling water to top off the jar.

4. Let the mixture steep for 20 minutes. Strain off and discard the herbs.

5. Soak a piece of cloth in the tea, gently squeeze it to remove the excess, and apply to the affected area. Leave on for 20 minutes.

TO USE: Repeat the application 2 to 3 times daily for 2 weeks. The tea can be reheated and used for up to 4 days. Store it in an airtight container in the refrigerator.

NOTE: Add this to a soaking bath to relieve vaginal yeast infections.

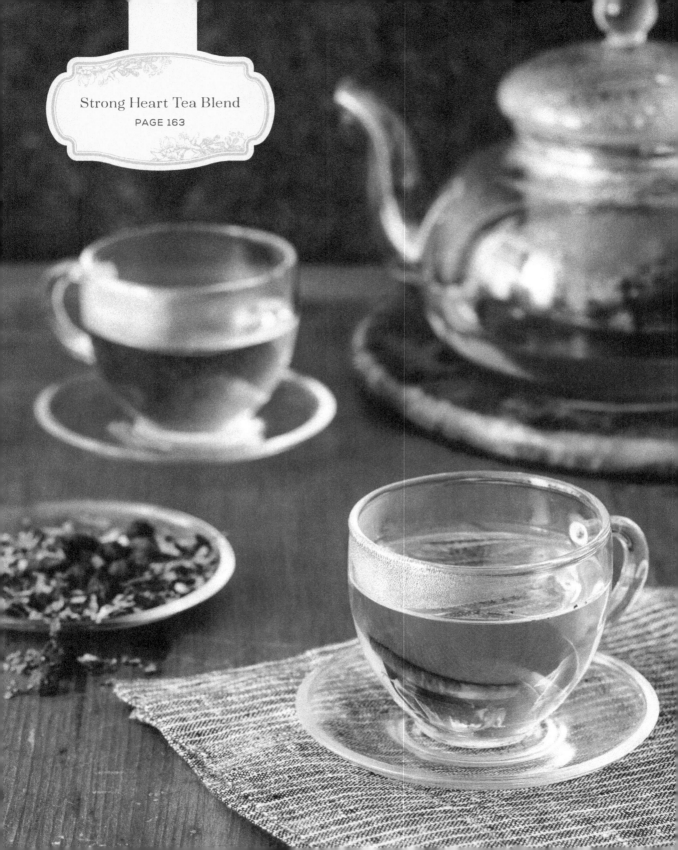

Strong Heart Tea Blend
PAGE 163

CHAPTER EIGHT

MEN'S HEALTH

Men have health needs specific to their bodies, just like women. In this chapter, I offer some recipes for health issues that are not gender specific but are more common in men, including heart disease and hair loss.

Most of the recipes in this chapter focus on men's reproductive health, with three focusing on prostate health. They include Benign Prostatic Hyperplasia Tonic (page 166), Prostatitis Formula (page 169), and Malignant Prostatic Enlargement Formula (page 170). Though these recipes should not be used in place of seeing a health care provider, they contain herbs that have been proven to support prostate health, reduce swelling in the prostate, and ease symptoms such as frequent urination.

In addition, I also provide several recipes to support penis health and general virility, along with a powder blend to help reduce and prevent chafing.

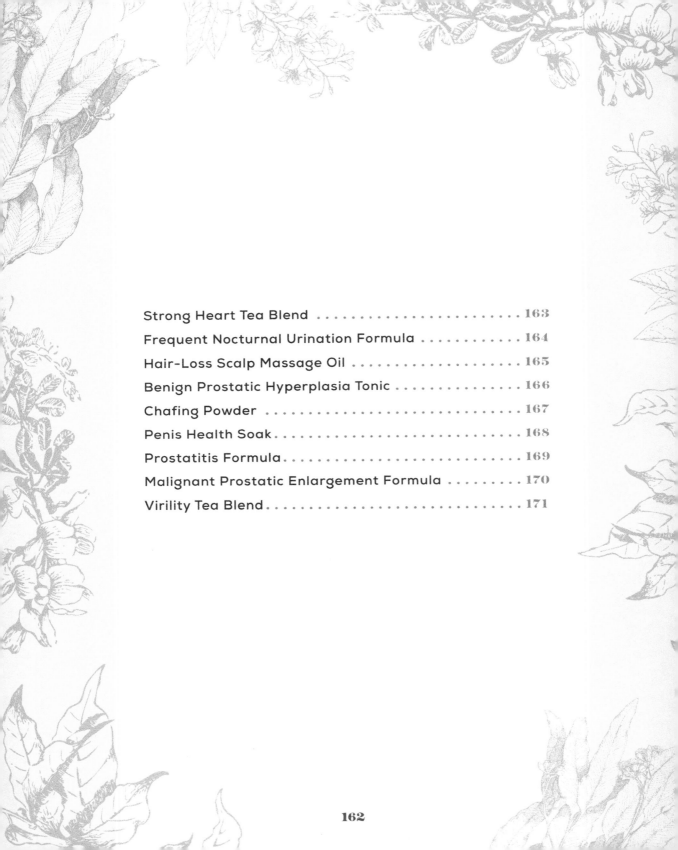

STRONG HEART TEA BLEND

As we age, it's important to keep our heart muscles strong and healthy. These herbs are great for strengthening the heart, relieving heart palpitations and rapid heart rate, and protecting the heart emotionally. The flavor is mildly sweet from the berries with a bit of sharpness, similar to black tea. Take this formula regularly and be sure to express your feelings, take time to enjoy life, eat healthy food, drink plenty of water, and reject violence in your life. If you are a woman reading this, support the men in your life by encouraging them to follow these suggestions.

Combine all the ingredients, and store in an airtight container. Label with the list of ingredients, date, and instructions for use.

TO USE: Steep 1 tablespoon of the tea blend in 10 ounces of boiling water for 15 to 20 minutes. Drink 1 to 2 cups daily.

NOTE: If you have a heart condition, be sure to consult your health care practitioner. See also the Heartbreak Tea Blend (page 113) and the Heart Health Tea Blend (page 186).

Makes enough for 24 cups of tea

½ cup hawthorn berries
½ cup dried hawthorn leaves and flowers
¼ cup dried motherwort
¼ cup dried ground ivy

FREQUENT NOCTURNAL URINATION FORMULA

A swollen prostate can cause frequent nocturnal urination because it presses against the urethra, blocking urine flow. This formula helps reduce swelling. It also supports muscles and nerves surrounding the prostate and bladder to help your body fully release urine from the bladder.

1. Add the tinctures to a 1-cup glass measuring cup and stir to combine.

2. Pour the mixture into a 4-ounce glass dropper bottle.

3. Tighten the dropper lid on the bottle, then label with the list of ingredients, date, and instructions for use.

TO USE: Add 30 drops of tincture to a small glass of water or juice, and drink 3 times daily.

NOTE: Use with the Benign Prostatic Hyperplasia Tonic (page 166) for best results.

Makes 4 ounces

2 ounces saw palmetto tincture
1 ounce St. John's wort tincture
1 ounce California poppy tincture

HAIR-LOSS SCALP MASSAGE OIL

Our hair starts to naturally thin as we age. These herbs help stimulate hair follicles and encourage hair growth. Choose a lighter oil such as sweet almond when infusing the herbs, or try apricot kernel for a less greasy massage oil.

1. Combine the oils together in a glass measuring cup and stir to combine.

2. Pour into an 8-ounce bottle.

3. Tighten the lid on the bottle, then label with the list of ingredients, date, and instructions for use. Store in the refrigerator, and discard at the first sign of rancidity.

TO USE: Massage into the scalp daily. Leave on for at least 8 hours for best results.

NOTE: Since this can make your hair look greasy, try applying before bedtime and rinsing it out in the morning.

Makes 8 ounces

2 ounces saw palmetto–infused oil

2 ounces stinging nettle leaf–infused oil

2 ounces rosemary-infused oil

2 ounces burdock seed–infused oil

BENIGN PROSTATIC HYPERPLASIA TONIC

Though this condition is not dangerous, it can lead to interrupted sleep due to frequent urination and urinary tract infections. More advanced stages of the condition can cause additional issues with the bladder and kidneys. The herbs in this formula help shrink the prostate, increase the urine flow to help fully empty the bladder, and reduce inflammation.

1. Add the tinctures to a 1-cup glass measuring cup and stir to combine.

2. Pour the mixture into an 8-ounce glass dropper bottle.

3. Tighten the dropper lid on the bottle, then label with the list of ingredients, date, and instructions for use.

Makes 8 ounces

3 ounces stinging nettle seed tincture

2 ounces saw palmetto tincture

2 ounces vitex tincture

1 ounce plantain tincture

TO USE: Add 60 to 80 drops of tincture to a small glass of water or juice, and drink 3 to 4 times daily. Take daily for up to 6 months.

NOTE: Try to avoid heavy consumption of coffee, alcohol, amphetamines, and antihistamines, which can increase symptoms.

CHAFING POWDER

Chafing is irritation caused by repetitive skin-to-skin friction in the thighs, armpits, and testicles, among other areas. The affected areas become sore, inflamed, and may burn. This powder helps prevent chafing, reduce moisture, and soothe irritation.

1. Mix the powdered herbs and arrowroot in a bowl and stir to combine.

2. Pour into a container with a shaker lid. Label with the list of ingredients, date, and instructions for use.

TO USE: Apply as needed.

NOTE: This recipe can be doubled. To increase absorbency, add ¼ cup bentonite clay to the blend.

Makes 1½ cups

¼ cup powdered calendula

¼ cup powdered gotu kola

1 tablespoon powdered comfrey root

1 cup arrowroot powder

PENIS HEALTH SOAK

This soak is a great way to help reduce itching, irritation, redness, and mild infections of the penis. Little boys, who often get irritated penises, may giggle at the idea of sitting and soaking their penises, but this soak offers fairly rapid relief.

Combine all the ingredients, and store in an airtight container. Label with the list of ingredients, date, and instructions for use.

TO USE: Steep 1 tablespoon tea blend in 12 ounces of boiling water for 10 to 15 minutes. Once it is cool enough to use comfortably, pour into a wide-mouth jar or bowl. For boys, a 4-ounce jelly jar works great. For teens and men, a wide-mouth 8-ounce canning jar or a bowl will work well. They should sit naked from the waist down on the floor in a comfortable location and rest their penis (with or without the testicles) in the warm soak for 10 to 15 minutes. Repeat 2 to 3 times daily until all signs of irritation are gone.

NOTE: Uncircumcised males should gently retract the foreskin of their penises while soaking.

Makes 6 cups

1½ tablespoons dried rosemary

1½ tablespoons dried thyme

1 tablespoon dried blackberry leaves

1 tablespoon dried prunella

1 tablespoon dried yarrow

1 teaspoon sea salt

PROSTATITIS FORMULA

Prostatitis is the inflammation or infection of the prostate. This also can affect the urinary tract and bladder. Symptoms include an aching pain in the area of the prostate, pain when sitting, difficulty urinating and draining the bladder, frequent dribbling, and sometimes chills, fever, and blood in the urine. Use these herbs to help clear up prostatitis, and be sure to follow up with a health care provider if this condition is suspected.

1. Add the tinctures to a 1-cup glass measuring cup and stir to combine.

2. Pour the mixture into an 8-ounce glass dropper bottle.

3. Tighten the dropper lid on the bottle, then label with the list of ingredients, date, and instructions for use.

TO USE: Add 25 to 40 drops of tincture to a small glass of water or juice, and drink 3 to 4 times daily. Continue taking for 2 days after symptoms disappear.

NOTE: Use a firm seat (no cushions on chairs), drink plenty of water, avoid long rides in vehicles or on bicycles, reduce your use of alcohol, caffeine, and hot, spicy food, and avoid sexual intimacy. Urinate frequently to avoid adding pressure on the prostate.

Makes 8 ounces

2 ounces saw palmetto tincture

2 ounces spilanthes tincture

1 ounce prunella tincture

1 ounce vitex tincture

1 ounce yarrow tincture

1 ounce stinging nettle leaf tincture

MALIGNANT PROSTATIC ENLARGEMENT FORMULA

Cancer in any form can be scary, but thankfully, prostate cancer is particularly slow growing. There are two forms of prostate cancer, the localized form and the advanced form. The localized form is the most common type and can often be managed with herbs. Reishi is a medicinal mushroom that is excellent at suppressing cancer cells, and stinging nettle root and saw palmetto have properties that are especially useful for addressing prostate issues. Always work with a health care practitioner in conjunction with herbal care for cancer. Herbalist James Green has a great book on men's health, and if you or a loved one is facing MPE, I highly recommend reading his thoughts on the topic. (See the Resources section on page 227 for more information.)

Makes 8 ounces

4 ounces reishi tincture

2 ounces saw palmetto tincture

2 ounces stinging nettle root tincture

1. Add the tinctures to a 1-cup glass measuring cup and stir to combine.

2. Pour the mixture into an 8-ounce glass dropper bottle.

3. Tighten the dropper lid on the bottle, then label with the list of ingredients, date, and instructions for use.

TO USE: Add 60 drops of tincture to a small glass of water or juice, and drink 3 times daily in a small glass of water for 6 months or longer.

NOTE: It is important to follow a whole food diet, get plenty of rest and exercise, and focus on being as stress free as possible during a cancer protocol. Seek out meditation, yoga, or another form of a stress-reduction practice to help maintain a positive mind-set throughout the protocol.

VIRILITY TEA BLEND

Impotence can be caused by a number of things, and, like many health issues, it cannot be healed by herbs alone. It can be a sign of an emotional imbalance, poor circulation, a weak immune system, stress, or endocrine system problems. Work with a health care practitioner to find the cause, and add this tea to your treatment plan to help support the endocrine, nervous, circulatory, and reproductive systems.

Combine all the ingredients in an airtight container. Label with the list of ingredients, date, and instructions for use.

TO USE: Steep 2 to 3 teaspoons of the tea blend in 8 ounces of boiling water for 25 to 30 minutes. You may wish to add honey to sweeten your tea. Drink 2 to 3 cups daily.

NOTE: Queen Anne's lace is wild carrot. If you can't find a source for Queen Anne's lace, add carrots to your daily diet for similar effects.

Makes enough for 20 to 30 cups of tea

¼ cup dried hawthorn leaves and flowers

¼ cup dried milky oats

¼ cup dried reishi

¼ cup dried stinging nettle leaves

2 tablespoons dried burdock root

2 tablespoons dried Queen Anne's lace seeds

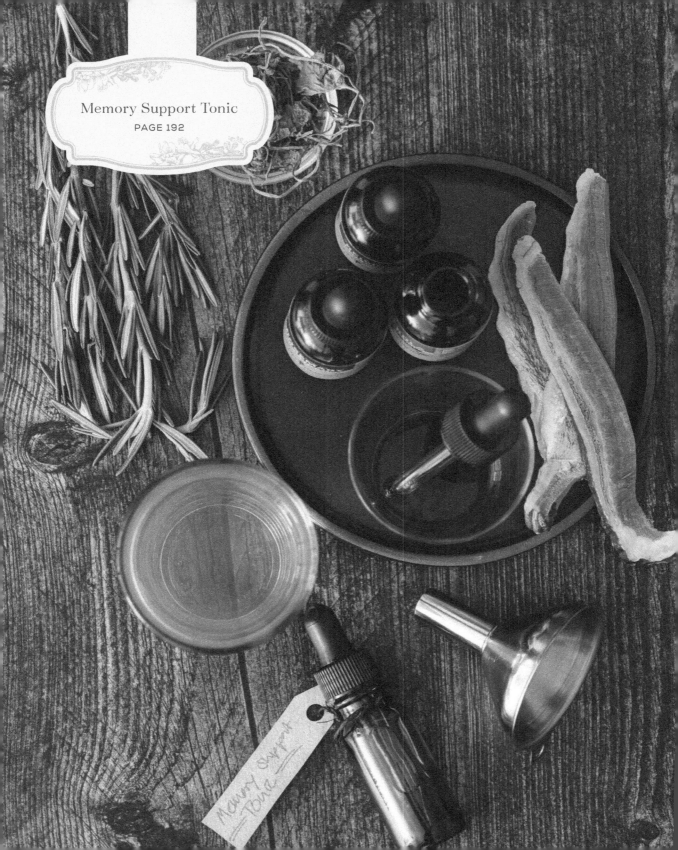

Memory Support Tonic
PAGE 192

CHAPTER NINE

AGING

As we grow older, our bodies begin to change. We lose natural elasticity in the skin, age spots start to appear, digestive issues start to surface (from acid reflux to a decreased ability to process sugars) circulatory issues start to rise (from high blood pressure to varicose veins), and our hearing and vision start to fail. Even our memory seems to leave us when we leave a room.

Though we can't stop the aging process, herbs are really good for helping to soften the symptoms. In this chapter, you'll find recipes that cover circulatory health, such as the Hypertension Formula (page 187), Cholesterol-Lowering Tonic (page 180), and Varicose Vein and Hemorrhoid Spray (page 197).

For musculoskeletal and nervous system issues, there are recipes such as Arthritis and Gout Cream (page 177), Plantar Fasciitis Salve (page 193), and Restless Leg Support Formula (page 194).

If you need help with your vision or hearing, look for the Eye Health Tonic Wash (page 183), Hearing Loss Tea Blend (page 185), and Tinnitus Tamer Tonic (page 196).

These recipes will help you tackle your specific needs as you move into middle age and beyond, so you can grow old gracefully with herbal support.

ACID REFLUX FORMULA

Many people think acid reflux is caused by too much acid in the stomach, but it is actually a result of your body producing too little acid during the early stages of digestion. To make up for the lack of acid, your body begins producing acid at a faster rate than normal, causing the reflux, which is sometimes referred to as heartburn. The best way to correct this is to introduce bitters into our system before we eat to stimulate digestion, which will get our stomach juices flowing in time to greet our food and digest it. We can do this by taking bitters about 20 minutes before a meal. As the name implies, they are bitter in taste. Do not sweeten this formula with honey; you need to taste the bitter for the herbs to do their job and stimulate the digestive process.

1. Add the tinctures to a 1-cup glass measuring cup and stir to combine.

2. Pour the mixture into an 8-ounce glass dropper bottle.

3. Tighten the dropper lid on the bottle, then label with the list of ingredients, date, and instructions for use.

TO USE: Swallow 30 to 60 drops about 20 minutes before a meal.

NOTE: This formula also can be made with apple cider vinegar instead of alcohol. Follow the instructions for making an acetum (page 62), and take the same dosage amount.

Makes 8 ounces

2 ounces dandelion leaf tincture

2 ounces burdock root tincture

1 ounce motherwort tincture

1 ounce black haw tincture

1 ounce catnip tincture

1 ounce mugwort tincture

AGE SPOTS FADE CREAM

Age spots, often referred to as liver spots, are dark skin pigmentations that appear on the skin due to exposure to the sun. This recipe is based off of a salve recipe I used to sell at my local farmer's market as a general wound salve. One of my customers noticed that it cleared up her age spots, and she was thrilled to show me the results.

1. Follow the instructions on page 70 to make a cream.

2. Pour your cream into an 8-ounce wide-mouth jar. Label with the list of ingredients, date, and instructions for use, and store in a cool location.

TO USE: Apply to skin pigmentation 2 to 3 times daily.

NOTE: This also can be simplified into an infused oil by simply omitting the tea, decoction, and borax.

Makes 8 ounces

2 ounces calendula-infused oil

2 ounces comfrey root–infused oil

2 ounces calendula tea

2 ounces comfrey root decoction

¼ ounce beeswax

½ teaspoon borax

ARTHRITIS AND GOUT CREAM

Arthritis and gout are two conditions that cause inflammation of the joints. When joints become inflamed, they become red, tender, stiff, and swollen. The herbs in this cream help relieve pain and inflammation.

1. Follow the instructions on page 70 to make a cream.

2. Pour your cream into an 8-ounce wide-mouth jar. Label with the list of ingredients, date, and instructions for use, and store in a cool location.

TO USE: Apply to achy joints 2 to 3 times daily.

NOTE: The sting in stinging nettles is often employed as an old-time arthritis remedy, known as uritification. If you have a patch of stinging nettles and are brave, you can try brushing against them to get stung on any achy joints. I can vouch firsthand that it worked for me. Also, consuming stinging nettle infusions 3 to 4 times weekly (see how to make infusions in chapter 3, page 61) can be of help.

Makes 8 ounces

2 ounces dried mugwort tea

2 ounces dried yarrow tea

2 ounces plantain-infused oil

2 ounces rosemary root–infused oil

¼ ounce beeswax

½ teaspoon borax

BROKEN-BONE-SUPPORT TEA BLEND AND COMPRESS

When we think of broken bones, we often picture a bone snapped in two, but breaks often are small fractures or cracks. Symptoms include swelling, pain, and skin bruising around the area of the break. Bones generally heal in 4 to 6 weeks, and a diet high in protein, calcium, and magnesium helps the recovery process. Another way to speed recovery is by taking herbs internally and applying this compress over the location of the break, if possible.

1. Combine the herbs in a bowl and stir to blend. Store in a half gallon jar. Label with the list of ingredients, date, and instructions for use.

2. To make your tea and compress, boil 1 quart of water.

3. If using the same blend internally and externally, add ½ cup to a quart jar and pour boiling water to top off jar.

4. Let steep for 20 minutes. Strain off the herbs and compost.

Makes enough for 14 cups of tea

2 cups dried blackberry leaves

2 cups dried milky oats

2 cups dried stinging nettle leaves

1 cup dried comfrey leaves

TO USE: Drink 2 cups of the tea blend daily. For the compress, soak a piece of cloth in the tea blend, gently squeeze to remove the excess, and apply over the broken bone. Leave on for 20 minutes. Repeat the application 2 to 3 times daily for 2 weeks. The strained tea you have made for the external application can be reheated and used for up to 4 days. Be sure to store it in an airtight container in the fridge between uses.

NOTE: Bone breaks are best remedied with a diet high in protein, calcium, and magnesium, as well as an internal and external herbal regimen, consisting of both herbal teas and poultices or compresses, if possible.

If you are concerned about the pyrrolizidine alkaloids in comfrey leaves, divide the tea blend between 2 bowls—one for internal use and one for external use—omitting the comfrey leaves in the internal-use batch. If using separate blends for internal and external use, add ¼ cup to a pint jar for each blend and pour boiling water to top off. If you are creating separate internal/external blends, be sure to note the information on the label. For more about comfrey's concerns, please see its herbal profile on page 48.

CHOLESTEROL-LOWERING TONIC

High cholesterol is an indication of inflammation happening in the circulatory system, which can damage the blood vessels. This condition can be triggered by diet, stress, and/or sleep deprivation. While herbs can be helpful, dietary and lifestyle changes are essential for lasting health.

1. Add the tinctures to a 1-cup glass measuring cup and stir to combine.

2. Pour the mixture into an 8-ounce glass dropper bottle.

3. Tighten the dropper lid on the bottle, then label with the list of ingredients, date, and instructions for use.

TO USE: Add 30 to 40 drops of tincture to a small glass of water or juice, and drink 3 times daily.

NOTE: Adding at least 2 cloves of garlic to your daily diet is a great way to help lower your cholesterol.

Makes 8 ounces

4 ounces hawthorn tincture

1 ounce gotu kola tincture

1 ounce dandelion leaf tincture

1 ounce black walnut leaf tincture

1 ounce reishi tincture

DIABETES FORMULA

This formula is for individuals who have type 2 diabetes. When combined with dietary and lifestyle changes, including exercise, a reduction of stress, and restful sleep, this blend can help reduce the need for (but not replace) insulin. Work with a health care practitioner to closely monitor your blood glucose levels so your insulin dosage can be adjusted accordingly.

1. Add the tinctures to a 1-cup glass measuring cup and stir to combine.

2. Pour the mixture into an 8-ounce glass dropper bottle.

3. Tighten the dropper lid on the bottle, then label with the list of ingredients, date, and instructions for use.

TO USE: Add 30 to 60 drops of tincture to a small glass of water or juice and drink 3 times daily.

NOTE: Don't forget to drink lots of water and eat wholesome foods—mostly vegetables and protein with small amounts of complex carbohydrates.

Makes 8 ounces

2 ounces dandelion leaf tincture

2 ounces Queen Anne's lace tincture

1 ounce burdock root tincture

1 ounce ground ivy tincture

1 ounce stinging nettle seed tincture

1 ounce yarrow tincture

ENERGY BALLS

Sometimes we need a bit of a boost to get through the day. Coffee and energy drinks contain large amounts of caffeine, which can be damaging to our nervous system. Try these energy balls instead! Daily consumption will increase your overall energy levels.

1. Combine the powdered herbs in a bowl (except for the optional listed powders).

2. Add in the tahini, honey, and molasses and stir to combine.

3. If your mixture is overly sticky, add more powdered stinging nettle leaves to thicken it. If it is overly thick, add a bit more honey or molasses to thin it.

4. Roll the mixture into 1-inch balls.

5. Roll each ball in cocoa powder, powdered coconut, or powdered reishi, if using.

6. Place in a shallow container with a lid and store in the fridge.

TO USE: Eat 2 to 3 balls as needed for a boost of energy.

NOTE: The tahini can be swapped out for any kind of nut butter such as peanut, almond, cashew, or sunflower seed butter.

*Makes about
20 (1-inch) balls*

1 cup powdered stinging nettle leaves

1 cup powdered gotu kola

½ cup dried stinging nettle seeds

½ cup tahini

2 tablespoons powdered ginger

2 tablespoons powdered reishi

3 tablespoons honey

2 tablespoons blackstrap molasses

Cocoa powder, powdered coconut, or extra powdered reishi (optional)

EYE HEALTH TONIC WASH

As we age, our eyes produce fewer tears, causing them to weaken and dry out—and sometimes become itchy, burning, and red. This tonic wash moisturizes eyes while soothing and toning them.

Combine the herbs (not the salt) in an airtight container. Label with the list of ingredients, date, and instructions for use.

Makes enough for 25 cups

½ cup dried prunella

¼ cup dried ground ivy

2 tablespoons dried gotu kola

2 tablespoons dried Queen Anne's lace

1 teaspoon sea salt (per dose)

TO USE: Steep 2 teaspoons of the tea blend in 8 ounces of boiling water for 15 to 20 minutes. Add 1 teaspoon sea salt to the blend, stirring to dissolve. When cooled, strain the mixture through a fine-mesh sieve into an eye cup. Lean forward, placing the cup tightly against your eye with your eye open. Stand upright and flip back your head so you are looking up at the ceiling. Blink several times, then bend forward again. Repeat this with fresh tea on the other eye, if needed. Rinse the eyes 1 to 2 times daily. The tea can be refrigerated for 3 to 4 days.

NOTE: For extra eye strengthening, look for a Tibetan eye chart online. These can be printed and used to help exercise your eye muscles, helping to improve vision when done daily over time.

GALL BLADDER TEA BLEND

The gall bladder can become inflamed and irritated due to a diet high in refined fats and foods that trigger sensitivities and allergic reactions. This formula eases inflammation and aids in bile production when combined with a proper diet for gall bladder health. If you suspect a gall bladder issue, consult with a health care practitioner.

Combine all the ingredients in an airtight container. Label with the list of ingredients, date, and instructions for use.

Makes enough for 16 cups of tea

¼ cup dried dandelion root

¼ cup dried burdock seeds

2 tablespoons dried black haw

2 tablespoons dried Queen Anne's lace

2 tablespoons dried spearmint

2 tablespoons dried yarrow

TO USE: Steep 1 tablespoon of the tea blend in 10 ounces of boiling water for 25 to 30 minutes. Drink 1 cup daily for gall bladder support. For an acute episode, drink several cups of tea throughout the day.

NOTE: Garlic and rosemary stimulate the gall bladder and can be added to your meals. Avoid sweets, rich food, greasy food, and any suspected allergen foods (corn, dairy, gluten, nightshades, shellfish, or yeast) if you are having gall bladder issues.

HEARING LOSS TEA BLEND

Hearing loss is part of the natural aging process, though lifetime exposure to prolonged, loud noise can make it worse. Though this blend cannot completely recover your hearing, it can be helpful to repair some of the damage. The monarda gives this tea some spice to round out the minty flavor of the ground ivy.

Combine all the ingredients in an airtight container. Label with the list of ingredients, date, and instructions for use.

TO USE: Steep 2 teaspoons of the tea blend in 8 ounces of boiling water for 15 to 20 minutes. Drink as needed.

NOTE: If you suffer from tinnitus without hearing loss, try the Tinnitus Tamer Tonic (page 196) instead of this formula.

Makes enough for 33 cups of tea

½ cup dried California poppy

½ cup dried ground ivy

¼ cup dried monarda

2 tablespoons dried plantain

HEART HEALTH TEA BLEND

Processed foods, stress, lack of exercise, high alcohol consumption, smoking, and obesity all contribute to heart disease. While herbs alone cannot heal heart disease, they can go a long way toward helping to strengthen and tone the heart and easing heart palpitations, rapid heart rate, and other heart irregularities. The herbs in this tea blend supplement dietary and lifestyle changes to support heart health.

Combine all the ingredients in an airtight container. Label with the list of ingredients, date, and instructions for use.

TO USE: Steep 2 teaspoons of the tea blend in 8 ounces of boiling water for 15 to 20 minutes. Drink as needed.

NOTE: If you are suffering from hypertension, see the Hypertension Formula (page 187). If you have any heart conditions, work with a health care practitioner to rule out any underlying health issues and monitor your heart while using this formula.

Makes enough for 21 cups of tea

¼ cup hawthorn berries

¼ cup dried hawthorn leaves and flowers

3 tablespoons dried motherwort

2 tablespoons dried ground ivy

1 tablespoon dried black haw

HYPERTENSION FORMULA

Hypertension can be reversible with dietary and lifestyle changes and a good herbal support system. This combination of herbs reduces fluid in the kidneys, dilates blood vessels, and increases circulation. It also supports venous integrity and strengthens the heart, helping to reduce blood pressure.

1. Add the tinctures to a 1-cup glass measuring cup and stir to combine.

2. Pour the mixture into an 8-ounce glass dropper bottle.

3. Tighten the dropper lid on the bottle, then label with the list of ingredients, date, and instructions for use.

TO USE: Add 30 drops of tincture to a small glass of water or juice and drink 3 times daily.

NOTE: This formula can be combined with the Cholesterol-Lowering Tonic (page 180) if you also are struggling with high cholesterol. If you are working to lower your blood pressure, be sure to monitor your blood pressure twice daily, and work with a health care practitioner to adjust any medications that you may be on.

Makes 8 ounces

2 ounces dandelion leaf tincture

1 ounce black haw tincture

1 ounce California poppy tincture

½ ounce hawthorn berry tincture

½ ounce dried hawthorn leaf and flower tincture

1 ounce ginger tincture

1 ounce reishi tincture

1 ounce yarrow tincture

HYPERTHYROID FORMULA

Hyperthyroidism can be an indication of a deeper condition, such as type 1 diabetes, Graves' disease, or Plummer disease. Symptoms such as unexplained weight loss, an irregular and/or rapid heartbeat, heart palpitations, tremors, sweating, increased appetite, thinning skin, and brittle hair may indicate a hyper thyroid. Lemon balm and motherwort have been shown to calm overactive thyroids, but be sure to work with a health care practitioner when dealing with thyroid issues.

1. Add the tinctures to a 1-cup glass measuring cup and stir to combine.

2. Pour the mixture into a 4-ounce glass dropper bottle.

3. Tighten the dropper lid on the bottle, then label with the list of ingredients, date, and instructions for use.

Makes 4 ounces

2 ounces lemon balm tincture
2 ounces motherwort tincture

TO USE: Add 30 to 60 drops of tincture to a small glass of water or juice and drink 3 times daily.

NOTE: If you suspect a thyroid issue, limit your intake of foods that contain iodized salt, seafood, seaweed, processed meats, and refined foods (sugar, pasta, white bread), as well as processed and deep-fried foods and caffeinated beverages.

HYPOTHYROID FORMULA

When you are diagnosed with hypothyroidism, it means that your thyroid isn't producing enough hormones. Symptoms include fatigue, sensitivity to cold, muscle weakness, elevated blood cholesterol levels, dry skin, unexplained weight gain, constipation, enlarged thyroid gland, and depression, among others. The stinging nettles and black walnut in this formula work great to treat a sluggish thyroid and goiters.

1. Add the tinctures to a 1-cup glass measuring cup and stir to combine.

2. Pour the mixture into a 4-ounce glass dropper bottle.

3. Tighten the dropper lid on the bottle, then label with the list of ingredients, date, and instructions for use.

Makes 4 ounces

2 ounces rotten (black) walnut hull tincture

2 ounces stinging nettle leaf tincture

TO USE: Add 30 to 60 drops of tincture to a small glass of water or juice and drink 3 times daily.

NOTE: If you're making your own tincture, be sure to collect the walnut hulls after they've turned black. For an underactive thyroid, also include seaweed and other foods rich in iodine, such as eggs and fish, in your diet.

KIDNEY SUPPORT TONIC

This formula combines herbs to offer kidney support and improve function. Regular use of this formula, and especially stinging nettle seed tincture, can help prevent or slow down renal failure when caught in the early stages.

1. Add the tinctures to a 1-cup glass measuring cup and stir to combine.

2. Pour the mixture into an 8-ounce glass dropper bottle.

3. Tighten the dropper lid on the bottle, then label with the list of ingredients, date, and instructions for use.

Makes 8 ounces

2 ounces Queen Anne's lace tincture

2 ounces stinging nettle seed tincture

1 ounce blackberry leaf tincture

1 ounce ground ivy tincture

TO USE: Add 30 to 60 drops of tincture to a small glass of water or juice and drink 3 times daily.

NOTE: Work with a health care practitioner to regulate kidney function, and follow an appropriate diet while using this tonic.

LIVER SUPPORT DECOCTION BLEND

The liver helps to rid the body of toxins that we ingest every day through our diet and chemical-based health care products, including medications. But over time, the liver can become overloaded. This decoction helps to support, tone, and detoxify the liver, improving its functionality.

Combine all the ingredients in an airtight container. Label with the list of ingredients, date, and instructions for use.

TO USE: Add 1 tablespoon of the decoction to a saucepan with 12 ounces of water. Bring to a boil, and then turn down and simmer for 15 to 20 minutes. Sweeten with honey and milk of your choice. Drink 1 to 2 cups daily.

NOTE: You may wish to add chai spices to this blend to enhance the flavor. Play around with a few tablespoons each of broken cinnamon sticks, cardamom pods, whole black peppercorns, and anise seed.

Makes enough for 17 cups of tea

½ cup dried dandelion root

¼ cup dried blackberry root

2 tablespoons dried burdock root

2 tablespoons dried yellow dock root

1 tablespoon dried ginger

MEMORY SUPPORT TONIC

Brain fog, forgetfulness, lack of concentration—these happen to all of us as we age. Memory loss occurs for a variety of reasons, including decreased flow of blood to the brain, hormonal changes, and the deterioration of our hippocampus. Gotu kola and rosemary both stimulate the brain, enhancing our mental abilities. Reishi, in particular, is an adaptogen and improves energy, focus, and calm to reduce mental and physical stress.

1. Add the tinctures to a 1-cup glass measuring cup and stir to combine.

2. Pour the mixture into a 4-ounce glass dropper bottle.

3. Tighten the dropper lid on the bottle, then label with the list of ingredients, date, and instructions for use.

Makes 4 ounces

2 ounces gotu kola tincture
1 ounce reishi tincture
1 ounce rosemary tincture

TO USE: Add 30 to 60 drops of tincture to a small glass of water or juice and drink 3 times daily.

NOTE: The longer you take the formula, the more you'll notice improved memory function. You may not notice a huge change at first, but eventually you'll find you can remember more and more little things you used to forget, like why you walked into a room or what you needed to purchase at the store.

PLANTAR FASCIITIS SALVE

Plantar fasciitis is a type of inflammation that appears on the bottom of your feet. It's often worse in the morning when you wake up, or after you've been standing for a long time. This blend of herbs fights inflammation and can provide healing and relief from the pain.

1. Follow the instructions on page 68 to make a salve.

2. Label with the list of ingredients, date, and instructions for use.

TO USE: Apply a small amount of salve to the affected area and massage. Reapply every 4 to 6 hours, as needed.

NOTE: Bring an extra pair of shoes with you so you can change footwear if your feet start hurting. It also helps to wear only shoes without heels. For additional relief, try rolling a tennis ball or foam roller on the floor with your bare feet.

Makes 4 ounces

1 ounce calendula-infused oil

1 ounce ginger-infused oil

1 ounce gotu kola–infused oil

½ ounce black haw–infused oil

½ ounce beeswax

1 vitamin E gelcap

RESTLESS LEG SUPPORT FORMULA

Restless Leg Syndrome (RLS) is characterized by an uncontrollable urge to move your legs that generally worsens over time and in the evening. Milky oats help to calm the nervous system and nerves that can cause overactive twitching, while black haw helps to calm muscle spasms.

1. Add the tinctures to a 1-cup glass measuring cup and stir to combine.

2. Pour the mixture into a 4-ounce glass dropper bottle.

3. Tighten the dropper lid on the bottle, then label with the list of ingredients, date, and instructions for use.

Makes 4 ounces

3 ounces black haw tincture
1 ounce milky oat tincture

TO USE: Add 20 to 40 drops of tincture to a small glass of water or juice and drink 3 times daily. For acute episodes, increase to 4 to 5 times daily.

NOTE: Consider taking a magnesium citrate supplement before bed every night to help with restless legs. Epsom salt baths can be helpful, too. Work with your health care practitioner to rule out other conditions such as an iron or magnesium deficiency.

SHINGLES SUPPORT TEA BLEND

Shingles, or herpes zoster, is caused by the same virus as chickenpox. Typically, it presents as a painful skin rash with blisters in a wide strip on either side of the body. This formula helps to kill the virus and soothe itching and inflammation. For extra healing, use oatmeal baths and apply chamomile essential oil on the rashes for relief.

Combine all the herbs (not the tincture) in an airtight container. Label with the list of ingredients, date, and instructions for use.

TO USE: Steep 2 teaspoons of the tea blend in 8 ounces of boiling water for 15 to 20 minutes. Add 30 drops of St. John's wort tincture to the tea, and drink 3 to 4 cups daily.

NOTE: For extra support and relief, take this remedy with Chickenpox Elixir (page 126).

Makes enough for 25 cups of tea

½ cup dried prunella

¼ cup dried lemon balm

2 tablespoons dried wild cherry

2 tablespoons dried yarrow

1 tablespoon dried black walnut leaves

30 drops St. John's wort tincture (per dose)

TINNITUS TAMER TONIC

If you suffer from ringing, buzzing, chirping, hissing, whistling, or other sounds in your ears, chances are that you have tinnitus. Whether the noise is constant or intermittent, this herbal remedy helps reduce and may even eliminate the issue with regular use.

1. Add the tinctures to a 1-cup glass measuring cup and stir to combine.

2. Pour the mixture into a 2-ounce glass dropper bottle.

3. Tighten the dropper lid on the bottle, then label with the list of ingredients, date, and instructions for use.

Makes 2 ounces

1¾ ounces ground ivy leaf tincture
¼ ounce monarda tincture

TO USE: Add 30 to 60 drops of tincture to a small glass of water or juice and drink 3 times daily.

NOTE: It can take a few months of use for ground ivy to take effect, but monarda acts more quickly, often within days or weeks. If you suffer from hearing loss with tinnitus, try the Hearing Loss Tea Blend instead (page 185).

VARICOSE VEIN AND HEMORRHOID SPRAY

This spray soothes varicose veins and hemorrhoids, both of which are caused by a lack of circulation. These herbs help tone veins and stimulate the valves to function properly so blood flow improves.

1. Add the tinctures and water to a 1-cup glass measuring cup and stir to combine.

2. Pour the mixture into a 4-ounce glass bottle with a spray top lid.

3. Tighten the lid on the bottle, then label with the list of ingredients, date, and instructions for use.

Makes 4 ounces

1 ounce yarrow tincture
½ ounce black walnut leaf tincture
½ ounce calendula tincture
2 ounces distilled water

TO USE: Spray onto varicose veins or hemorrhoids 3 times daily. For acute episodes, increase to 4 to 5 times daily.

NOTE: This formula can be made into an oil or salve to be applied topically if you prefer an oil-based product. For best results, also make an additional tincture for internal use by eliminating the water and adding 2 ounces dried hawthorn leaves and flowers. Take 30 drops 3 times daily.

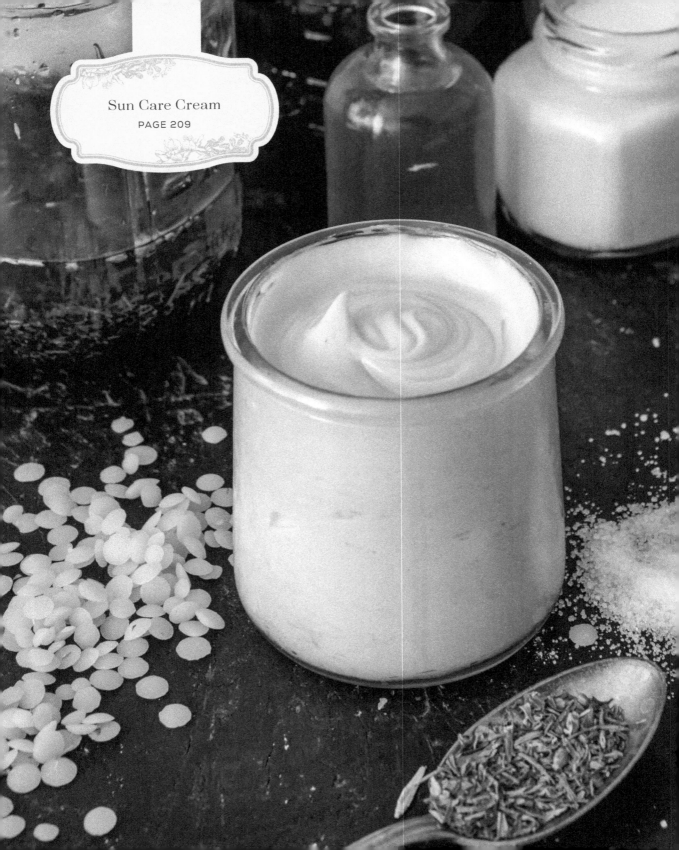

Sun Care Cream

PAGE 209

CHAPTER TEN

PERSONAL CARE

Herbal medicine isn't just for bumps and bruises and everyday ailments. Herbs also are ideal for personal care. From luxurious, relaxing baths to herbal hair rinses and fabulous facial cleaners, this section has a whole array of body care products you can easily make at home.

If you're looking for products to cover outdoor activities, check out the Sun Care Cream (page 209) and the Bug Repellant Spray (page 206).

Everyday hygiene is covered with recipes for Tooth-Cleansing Powder (page 220), Mouthwash (page 219), and Shaving Cream (page 204) as well as for Aftershave Toner (page 213) and Natural Cream Deodorant (page 207). Whether you have oily, dry, or combination skin, herbal face cleansers (pages 210 to 212) are provided for all skin types.

End your day in a relaxing bath with Bath Salts (page 202) or Bath Tea Blend (page 203) and a nourishing hair rinse based on your hair type (pages 215 to 217).

AFTER-BATH OIL

This oil nourishes and moisturizes skin and makes a great oil for applying after baths. Use almond oil for a lighter moisturizer, coconut oil for extra skin conditioning, or hemp seed oil for extra nourishment.

1. Pour the oils into a glass measuring cup and stir to combine. Empty the contents of the vitamin E gelcaps into the oil mixture and stir well.

2. Pour the mixture into an 8-ounce bottle. Tighten the lid, then label with the list of ingredients, date, and instructions for use.

TO USE: Apply to skin after bathing.

NOTE: If you'd like, you can add a scent with a few drops of essential oil. Calendula, lavender, rose geranium, or rock rose all make nice, aromatic additions to this blend.

Makes 8 ounces

2 ounces borage-infused oil

2 ounces prunella-infused oil

2 ounces calendula-infused oil

1 ounce gotu kola–infused oil

1 ounce plantain-infused oil

4 vitamin E gelcaps

BATH SALTS

Sometimes after a long day, a soak in the bath is just what's needed to help you relax. Baths salts are a great way to help draw out toxins from the skin, helping our body detox from illnesses and environmental toxins absorbed through the skin. They can be drying, however, so don't use them on a daily basis.

Combine all the ingredients in an airtight container. Label with the list of ingredients, date, and instructions for use.

TO USE: Add 1 cup of the bath salts to your bath as the water is running. Stir with your hand to help dissolve the salts. Luxuriate in your bath for 20 minutes.

NOTE: This bath is best enjoyed with scented candles as you lean back and relax. Follow up with After-Bath Oil (page 201) to nourish and moisturize your skin.

Makes enough for 9 baths

4 cups Epsom salts
3 cups sea salt
1 cup powdered goldenrod
1 cup powdered oatmeal

BATH TEA BLEND

A great alternative to adding bath salts to your bath is using a bath tea, which allows your skin to absorb the relaxing and healing properties of herbs. This is an all-purpose nourishing skin blend. Don't be afraid to use the herb profiles in this book to mix and match ingredients for a bath blend to suit your individual needs.

Combine all the ingredients in an airtight container. Label with the list of ingredients, date, and instructions for use.

TO USE: Follow the instructions on page 73 to make an herbal bath. Soak in your bath for 20 to 30 minutes.

NOTE: Goldenrod, prunella, comfrey leaves, and yarrow are just a few of the herbs that can be used in herbal baths.

Makes enough for 8 baths

1 cup dried goldenrod
1 cup dried calendula
1 cup dried plantain
1 cup dried prunella

SHAVING CREAM

This shaving cream can be applied to any area of the body for protecting and soothing skin. Calendula, prunella, and comfrey are nourishing skin herbs that heal small abrasions and scrapes that can occur during shaving. The powdered oatmeal and borax provide extra slip to help the razor glide more smoothly over the skin.

1. Follow the instructions on page 70 to make a cream (adding the powdered oatmeal to the oil mixture).

2. Pour your cream into an 8-ounce wide-mouth jar. Label with the list of ingredients, date, and instructions for use. Store in a cool location.

TO USE: Apply to the skin in a thin coat before shaving.

NOTE: Follow with Aftershave Toner (page 213) or After-Bath Oil (page 201).

Makes 8 ounces

2 ounces calendula-infused oil

2 ounces prunella-infused oil

1 tablespoon powdered oatmeal

4 ounces comfrey leaf tea

¼ ounce beeswax

½ teaspoon borax

ATHLETE'S FOOT SOAK

Athlete's foot is a fungus that sets in and can make one miserable with itching and burning. This formula helps to clear up the fungus with the help of antifungal herbs and apple cider vinegar, which also is antifungal. For convenience, purchase a plastic shoebox to store the soak in. It makes a great vessel for soaking your feet and it has a snap-on lid to keep the contents from spilling out. This solution makes one batch, which can be reused for the duration of application.

1. Combine the dried herbs in a bowl. If you are using St. John's wort tincture, leave it out until step 3.

2. Pour the vinegar into a saucepan and bring it to a boil over medium-high heat. Turn off the heat and add the dried herbs.

3. Cover the pan and let the mixture steep for 8 to 12 hours, then add in the St. John's wort tincture, if using.

4. Store in a sealed container. Label with the list of ingredients, date, and instructions for use.

TO USE: Soak both feet in the solution for 5 to 7 minutes daily for 2 to 3 months. If the fungus has cleared up before the 2-month mark, you can stop using the soak at 2 months. Discard the mixture after 3 months.

NOTE: Trim your nails short and keep trimmed short for the duration of the application.

Makes a 3-month supply

1 tablespoon dried black walnut leaves

1 tablespoon dried spearmint

1 tablespoon dried yellow dock root

1 tablespoon freshly dried St. John's wort or 90 drops St. John's wort tincture

4 cups apple cider vinegar

BUG REPELLANT SPRAY

Mosquitos and other biting insects can really ruin an enjoyable outdoor experience, but most commercial bug repellants contain toxic chemicals that you don't want to spray on yourself or your kids. Try this herbal blend instead.

1. Combine the tinctures and water in a 1-cup glass measuring container and stir to combine.

2. Pour the mixture into a 4-ounce glass bottle with a spray-top lid. Tighten the lid, then label with the list of ingredients, date, and instructions for use.

Makes 4 ounces

1 ounce yarrow tincture
1 ounce catnip tincture
1 ounce lemon balm tincture
1 ounce distilled water

TO USE: Spray on exposed skin before going outdoors. Reapply as needed.

NOTE: For extra protection, spray this formula on clothing and hair, too.

NATURAL CREAM DEODORANT

Commercial deodorants and antiperspirants contain aluminum, which has been linked to Alzheimer's and dementia. While you will still sweat with this deodorant, the ingredients help absorb it while killing the odor-causing bacteria. Best of all, this deodorant generally only needs one daily application to be effective.

1. Begin by infusing the thyme and rosemary in the coconut oil and shea butter, following instructions on page 66. Strain out the herbs and compost them.

2. Combine the arrowroot, bentonite, and baking soda in a bowl; set aside.

3. Place the oil in a mixing bowl and start to beat it with an electric mixer. With the mixer running, slowly start adding the powder mixture to the oils, about 2 to 3 tablespoons at a time. Continue mixing until all of the powder has been blended in.

4. Using a spatula or spoon, scrape your deodorant into a wide-mouth jar. Seal the lid, and label with the list of ingredients, date, and instructions for use.

Makes about 7 ounces

1 teaspoon dried thyme
1 teaspoon dried rosemary
3 tablespoons shea butter
2 tablespoons coconut oil
6 tablespoons
  arrowroot powder
2 tablespoons
  bentonite clay
1 tablespoon baking soda

TO USE: Pinch a pea-size piece of deodorant from the container, rub with your thumb and fingers to soften it, and then apply it directly to your pits.

NOTE: If you're sensitive to baking soda, omit it from the recipe and increase the amount of arrowroot powder. You may wish to add a few drops of essential oil to scent your deodorant.

SCAR REPAIR CREAM

Comfrey root helps break down scar tissue, and gotu kola rejuvenates the skin. This combination of herbs helps dissolves scar tissue and rebuild healthy tissue, all while calendula nourishes the skin.

1. Follow the instructions on page 70 to make a cream.

2. Pour your cream into an 8-ounce wide-mouth jar. Label with the list of ingredients, date, and instructions for use. Store in a cool location.

TO USE: Apply to scar tissue 2 to 3 times daily.

NOTE: Though this works best on fresh scars, this cream also will help lessen the appearance of old scars over time.

Makes 8 ounces

2 ounces gotu kola–infused oil

2 ounces comfrey root–infused oil

2 ounces calendula tea

2 ounces comfrey root decoction

¼ ounce beeswax

½ teaspoon borax

SUN CARE CREAM

This cream is great for soothing sun-drenched skin that is hot, dry, and burned. Sunflower oil and shea butter possess sunscreen capabilities. St. John's Wort does, too, so this cream can be used every day on faces, hands, and arms.

1. Follow the instructions on page 70 to make a cream.

2. Pour your cream into an 8-ounce wide-mouth jar. Label with the list of ingredients, date, and instructions for use. Store in a cool location.

TO USE: Apply to exposed skin daily before heading outside or after you've been in the sun.

NOTE: Simplify this formula and make an infused oil by omitting the tea, decoction, and borax.

Makes 8 ounces

2 ounces St. John's wort–infused oil, using half shea butter and half sunflower oil

2 ounces blackberry leaf and root–infused oil, using half shea butter and half sunflower oil

2 ounces St. John's wort tea

2 ounces blackberry root decoction

¼ ounce beeswax

½ teaspoon borax

FACE CLEANSER FOR ALL TYPES

Oil cleansers help gently lift dirt, sebum, and makeup from your face while leaving your skin feeling soft and smooth. This blend of herbs balances and works well for all types of skin, absorbing excess oil while moistening dry zones.

1. Follow the instructions on page 66 to make an infused oil.

2. Pour your oil into a 2-ounce dropper bottle. Tighten the lid on the bottle, then label with the list of ingredients, date, and instructions for use.

Makes 2 ounces

1¾ ounces sunflower oil
¼ ounce castor oil
1 teaspoon dried rosemary
1 teaspoon dried plantain
1 teaspoon dried prunella

TO USE: Apply a dropperful of oil (about 30 drops) to your face. Gently massage for 1 to 2 minutes. Use a washcloth to wipe off the oil.

NOTE: For extra-deep cleaning, apply the oil to your face, then soak a washcloth in hot water. Wring out the excess water and place the washcloth over your face for 1 to 2 minutes. Remove the washcloth and gently wipe off the oil.

FACE CLEANSER FOR DRY SKIN

Dry skin can be red, patchy, and flaky, and many cleansers contain a detergent base or alcohol that can further irritate it. This oil cleanser gently lifts dirt, sebum, and makeup from your face, and the additions of borage, plantain, and Queen Anne's lace nourish your skin and leave it soft and smooth.

Makes 2 ounces

1¾ ounces sunflower oil
¼ ounce castor oil
1 teaspoon dried
  borage flower
1 teaspoon dried plantain
1 teaspoon dried Queen
  Anne's lace flower

1. Follow the instructions on page 66 to make an infused oil.

2. Pour your oil into a 2-ounce dropper bottle. Tighten the lid on the bottle, then label with the list of ingredients, date, and instructions for use.

TO USE: Apply a dropperful of oil (about 30 drops) to your face. Gently massage for 1 to 2 minutes. Use a washcloth to wipe away the oil.

NOTE: For extra-deep cleaning, apply the oil to your face, then soak a washcloth in hot water. Wring out the excess water and place the washcloth over your face for 1 to 2 minutes. Remove the washcloth and gently wipe off the oil.

FACE CLEANSER FOR OILY SKIN

It may seem counterintuitive to put oil on oily skin, but it actually helps remove the oil already on your face. When skin is washed with water and other products that strip the skin of its natural oils, it reacts by increasing oil production and causing even more oiliness. Using oil for cleansing rebalances the skin.

1. Follow the instructions on page 66 to make an infused oil.

2. Pour your oil into a 2-ounce dropper bottle. Tighten the lid on the bottle, then label with the list of ingredients, date, and instructions for use.

TO USE: Apply a dropperful of oil (about 30 drops) to your face. Gently massage for 1 to 2 minutes. Use a washcloth to wipe away the oil.

NOTE: For extra-deep cleaning, apply the oil to your face, then soak a washcloth in hot water. Wring out the excess water and place the washcloth over your face for 1 to 2 minutes. Remove the washcloth and gently wipe off the oil.

Makes 2 ounces

1¾ ounces sunflower oil
¼ ounce castor oil
1½ teaspoons dried yarrow
1½ teaspoons dried
    blackberry leaves

AFTERSHAVE TONER

Cutting hair close to the skin exposes pores, leaving them prone to dirt and debris. Aftershaves help tighten and refine pores after shaving. These herbs refresh skin and also are antiseptic to protect against infection from any razor nicks.

1. Combine the tinctures and infusion in a 1-cup glass measuring container and stir to combine.

2. Pour the mixture into an 8-ounce glass bottle with a spray-top lid. Tighten the lid on the bottle, then label with the list of ingredients, date, and instructions for use.

TO USE: Shake well and spritz onto shaved areas.

NOTE: If the spray bottle doesn't apply enough toner, change the lid to a regular cap and pour a small amount of toner into your hands to apply.

Makes 8 ounces

2 ounces plantain tincture

2 ounces prunella tincture

2 ounces calendula tincture

½ ounce spearmint tincture

1½ ounces comfrey leaf infusion

BEARD OIL

The herbs and oils in this formula nourish beard hair and the skin under the beard, while also reducing itching and irritation. Hemp oil is full of nutrients that help grow stronger and healthier hair and allow beards to grow longer, plus it also moisturizes the hair and skin. Jojoba oil is actually a wax containing tocopherols that strengthen and enhance the beard's natural oils and decrease breakage. Stinging nettles strengthen and nourish hair, and burdock seed conditions and moisturizes the skin.

1. Combine the oils in a glass measuring cup and stir to combine.

2. Pour the mixture into an 8-ounce bottle, tighten the lid, then label with the list of ingredients, date, and instructions for use. Store the oil in the refrigerator, and discard it at the first sign of rancidity.

Makes 2 ounces

1 ounce stinging nettle–infused jojoba oil

1 ounce burdock seed–infused hemp seed oil

TO USE: Massage a few drops into the beard.

NOTE: If you would like to add scent to the beard oil, you can add a few drops of essential oil. Patchouli has a nice, earthy scent, while bay leaves and cloves are spicier.

HAIR RINSE FOR LIGHT/BLOND HAIR

Calendula and goldenrod lighten and brighten hair, softening it in the process. This is an effective, nourishing blend for light hair shades.

Combine all the ingredients, and store the mixture in an airtight container. Label with the list of ingredients, date, and instructions for use.

Makes enough for 12 rinses

1½ cups dried calendula
1½ cups dried goldenrod

TO USE: Steep 4 tablespoons of the tea blend in 16 ounces of boiling water for 3 hours. Strain. Hold your head over a sink or tub and pour a few ounces of the infusion over your head, allowing it to drain into the sink. Massage the infusion into your hair and scalp with your fingers, then repeat with another few ounces of the infusion. Follow with a cool water rinse, if you like.

NOTE: For an extra rinse, collect the infusion as it runs through your hair, and repeat the process of pouring and massaging it into your hair and scalp several times.

HAIR RINSE FOR DARK/GREYING HAIR

Rosemary is a hair tonic and conditioner that darkens hair, and burdock helps prevent dandruff. Stinging nettles also fight dandruff, and they also tone and condition dark hair shades.

Combine all the ingredients, and store the mixture in an airtight container. Label with the list of ingredients, date, and instructions for use.

Makes enough for 12 rinses

1 cup dried rosemary

1 cup dried burdock root

1 cup dried stinging
  nettle leaves

TO USE: Steep 4 tablespoons of the tea blend in 16 ounces of boiling water for 3 hours. Strain. Hold your head over a sink or tub and pour a few ounces of the infusion over your head, allowing it to drain into the sink. Massage the infusion into your hair and scalp with your fingers, then repeat with another few ounces of the infusion. Follow with a cool water rinse, if you like.

NOTE: For an extra rinse, collect the infusion as it runs through your hair, and repeat the process of pouring and massaging it into your hair and scalp several times.

HAIR RINSE FOR STRENGTHENING HAIR

Catnip strengthens hair, helping it grow while soothing scalp irritations. Stinging nettles tone and condition hair while preventing dandruff. Plantain nourishes and strengthens hair.

Combine all the ingredients, and store the mixture in an airtight container. Label with the list of ingredients, date, and instructions for use.

Makes enough for 12 rinses

1 cup dried stinging nettle leaves
1 cup dried catnip
1 cup dried plantain

TO USE: Steep 4 tablespoons of the tea blend in 16 ounces of boiling water for 3 hours. Strain. Hold your head over a sink or tub and pour a few ounces of the infusion over your head, allowing it to drain into the sink. Massage the infusion into your hair and scalp with your fingers, then repeat with another few ounces of the infusion. Follow with a cool water rinse, if you like.

NOTE: For an extra rinse, collect the infusion as it runs through your hair, and repeat the process of pouring and massaging it into your hair and scalp several times.

FEVER BLISTER LIP BALM

Spilanthes, prunella, and lemon balm work as antiviral herbs to fight the virus that causes unsightly and painful fever blisters. With regular use, this lip balm can help prevent fever blisters from forming. It also makes a nourishing and protective treatment for chapped lips.

1. Begin by infusing the spilanthes, prunella, and lemon balm in the almond and jojoba oils, following the instructions on page 66.

2. Combine the infused oils with the shea butter and beeswax in a double boiler. Heat until all of the solid materials have melted.

3. Turn off the heat, then stir in the honey and vitamin E oil.

4. Using a 1-cup glass measuring container, pour the lip balm into tubes.

5. Let the balm cool completely, then label with the list of ingredients, date, and instructions for use.

Makes about 18 tubes

1 tablespoon dried
   spilanthes
1 tablespoon dried prunella
1 tablespoon dried
   lemon balm
½ ounce almond oil
½ ounce jojoba oil
1 ounce shea butter
1 ounce beeswax
⅛ teaspoon honey
⅛ teaspoon vitamin E oil

TO USE: Apply several times daily, as needed. This lip balm can be used to prevent and heal fever blisters.

NOTE: You may find it easier to heat the oils and wax with a glass measuring cup set in a saucepan with a bit of water. Be sure to grab the handle with a hot pad to avoid burns!

MOUTHWASH

Commercial mouthwashes contain harmful chemicals, a high alcohol content, which can damage gum tissue, and a variety of sweeteners. This is a refreshing mouthwash that contains a significantly lower amount of alcohol and no sweeteners. It reduces the buildup of bacteria, tones and tightens gums, and heals weak, irritated, and bleeding gums.

1. Add the tinctures to a 1-cup glass measuring cup and stir to combine.

2. Pour the mixture into a 4-ounce glass dropper bottle.

3. Tighten the dropper lid on the bottle, then label with the list of ingredients, date, and instructions for use.

TO USE: Add 60 drops of tincture to a small cup, then add 2 tablespoons of water. Pour the wash into your mouth, swish for 1 to 2 minutes, and then spit it out.

NOTE: Use this after brushing your teeth. If you are experiencing tooth pain, add 2 ounces of California poppy to the blend. Swish it in your mouth first without diluting it with water, holding it near the affected tooth for 1 to 2 minutes.

Makes 4 ounces

2 ounces spearmint tincture
½ ounce plantain tincture
½ ounce prunella tincture
½ ounce spilanthes tincture
¼ ounce yarrow tincture
¼ ounce yellow dock tincture

TOOTH-CLEANSING POWDER

Toothpastes contain gentle abrasives to help remove stains and bacteria from the teeth. Unfortunately, they also contain harmful ingredients such as sodium lauryl sulfate, which has been linked to canker sores and tooth sensitivity. This tooth powder helps kill bacteria, brightens teeth, and leaves them feeling smooth.

1. Preheat the oven to 150°F.

2. Using a mortar and pestle, grind together the salt and thyme to make a powder.

3. Spread the mixture on a rimmed baking sheet and bake for 1 to 2 hours or until the thyme is fully dried.

4. Regrind the mixture with the mortar and pestle, adding the baking soda and mixing well.

5. Transfer the mixture to a jar or other airtight container. Label with the list of ingredients, date, and instructions for use.

Makes enough for 36 applications

¼ cup sea salt
¼ cup fresh thyme leaves
¼ cup baking soda

TO USE: Wet your toothbrush and dip it into the powder or sprinkle about 1 teaspoon of the powder onto the toothbrush. Brush as usual.

NOTE: If you would like extra whitening power, add ⅛ cup activated charcoal to the baking soda.

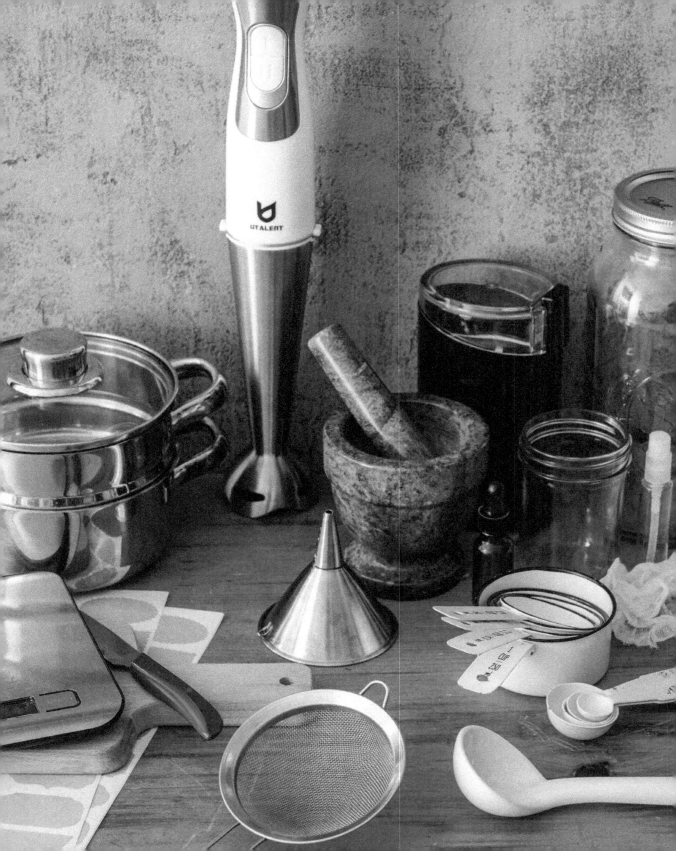

GLOSSARY

ACETUM: An herbal preparation made with herbs and vinegar

ADAPTOGEN: Helps balance; restores and protects the body

ADRENAL TONIC: Boosts the activity of the adrenal glands while toning and nourishing them

ALTERATIVE: Gradually restores healthy bodily functions (See also *depurative*)

ANABOLIC: The synthesis in living organisms of more complex substances from simpler ones

ANALGESIC: Reduces or eliminates pain without causing loss of consciousness

ANAPHRODISIAC: Suppresses libido

ANESTHETIC: Temporarily depresses neuronal function, producing total or partial loss of sensation

ANODYNE: Soothes or eliminates pain

ANTACID: Neutralizes stomach acidity

ANTHELMINTIC: Expels parasitic worms by stunning or killing them

ANTIALLERGENIC: Prevents or minimizes an allergic reaction

ANTIANDROGENIC: Inhibits the biological effects of androgens

ANTIBACTERIAL: Inhibits bacterial growth or kills bacteria

ANTIBIOTIC: Destroys or inhibits the growth of other microorganisms

ANTICATARRHAL: Helps remove excess mucus from the body

ANTIDEPRESSANT: Relieves depression and other mental conditions

ANTIDIARRHEAL: Provides symptomatic relief for diarrhea

ANTIEMETIC: Aids vomiting and nausea

ANTIESTROGENIC: Suppresses or inhibits estrogenic activity

ANTIFUNGAL: Inhibits fungal growth or kills fungi

ANTIHISTAMINE: Blocks histamine reactions

ANTI-INFLAMMATORY: Reduces inflammation

ANTILITHIC: Works against the formation of calculi, such as kidney stones

ANTIMALARIAL: Prevents or relieves malaria symptoms

ANTIMICROBIAL: Kills microorganisms or inhibits their growth

ANTIMUTAGENIC: Reduces or interferes with the mutagenic actions or effects of a substance

ANTINEOPLASTIC: Inhibits or prevents the growth or development of malignant cells

ANTIOXIDANT: Protects cells against the effects of free radicals

ANTIPARASITIC: Relieves parasitic diseases such as nematodes, cestodes, trematodes, and infectious protounceoa

ANTIRHEUMATIC: Alleviates or prevents rheumatism

ANTISCORBUTIC: Prevents or cures scurvy

ANTISEPTIC: Prevents infection by inhibiting the growth of microorganisms

ANTISPASMODIC: Relieves spasms

ANTITUMOR: Prevents or inhibits tumor formation or growth

ANTITUSSIVE: Suppresses coughs

ANTIVENOMOUS: Neutralizes venom

ANTIVIRAL: Inhibits viral growth or kills viruses

ANXIOLYTIC: Helps reduce or prevent anxiety

APERIENT: Has a mild purgative or laxative effect (See also *laxative*)

APHRODISIAC: Elevates, nourishes, and/or sustains intimacy and sensual desire

APPETITE STIMULANT: Stimulates the appetite

AROMATIC: Plants with high volatile oil levels that smell strongly and can stimulate the digestive system

ASTRINGENT: Tends to shrink or constrict body tissues

BIOGENIC STIMULATOR: Stimulates the metabolism, which activates the body's protective and regenerative functions

BITTER: Having or being a taste that is sharp, acrid, and unpleasant; not sweet, salty, or sour

BLOOD TONIC: Invigorates and nourishes blood; reinforces the effects of iron and other nutrients

BRAIN TONIC: Tonifies and supports the brain

BRONCHODILATOR: Dilates the bronchi and bronchioles, decreasing resistance in the respiratory airway and increasing airflow to the lungs (Also referred to as *bronchial dilators*)

CALMATIVE: Has a soothing effect

CARDIOTONIC: Acts as a tonic to the heart, toning the muscle and its action

CARMINATIVE: Induces gas expulsion from the stomach and intestines

CATHARTIC: Has purgative action

CEPHALIC: Has an effect on the head

CEREBRAL VASORELAXANT: Causes a decrease in vascular pressure, resulting in the reduction in tension of blood vessel walls in the brain

CHOLAGOGUE: Supports the gall bladder and liver by promoting the flow of bile from the gall bladder into the intestines

CHOLERETIC: Increases the volume of secretion of bile from the liver and the amount of solids secreted

CIRCULATORY STIMULANT: Promotes better circulation of blood from the trunk of the body to the periphery, warming tissues, particularly in the hands and feet

COMPRESS: A piece of cloth soaked in a tea or infusion of herbs and applied to the affected area of the body

CONTRACEPTIVE: Prevents pregnancy

DECOCTION: A tea-like drink of herbs produced by boiling them in water; generally made from roots, bark, and seeds

DECONGESTANT: Helps relieve nasal congestion in the upper respiratory tract

DEMULCENT: Forms a soothing film over mucous membranes to relieve pain and minor inflammation of that area

DEOBSTRUENT: Clears or opens natural ducts in the body (removes obstructions)

DEPURATIVE: Purifies or works as a purgative for the blood (See also *alterative*)

DETOXIFIER: Counteracts or destroys toxic properties

DIAPHORETIC: Promotes sweating, helping relieve a fever through perspiration

DIFFUSION: The movement of a substance from an area of higher concentration to an area of lower concentration (Another name for *tea* or *tisane*)

DIGESTIVE: Aids digestion

DISCUTIENT: An agent or process that disperses a tumor or lesion

DISINFECTANT: Destroys bacteria

DIURETIC: Stimulates urine flow

DOUBLE EXTRACTION: An herbal preparation made by extracting and preserving the active properties of herbs by first using alcohol, then adding the strained herbs to water to create a decoction. Once these steps have been taken, the alcohol extract and water decoction are combined

EMETIC: Causes vomiting

EMMENAGOGUE: Stimulates blood flow in the pelvic area, which can bring on menstruation

EMOLLIENT: Soothes and protects the skin when applied externally; heals inflamed or irritated mucous membranes when taken internally

ENDOCRINE TONIC: Restores balance to the endocrine system

ESTROGENIC: Promotes or produces estrus

EUPHORIANT: Induces a feeling of euphoria

EXPECTORANT: Promotes and facilitates the discharge of mucus and fluids from the respiratory tract

FEBRIFUGE: Reduces fever

GALACTAGOGUE: Increases milk supply during lactation

HEMOSTATIC: Works to slow or stop bleeding or hemorrhaging

HEPATIC: Acts on the liver

HEPATOPROTECTIVE: Protects and prevents damage to the liver

HYPERTENSIVE: Increases blood pressure

HYPNOTIC: Calming to the point of inducing sleep

HYPOCHOLESTEROLEMIC: Facilitates the lowering of cholesterol in the body

HYPOGLYCEMIC: Lowers glucose levels in the blood

HYPOTENSIVE: Reduces blood pressure

IMMUNE TONIC: Helps nourish, tone, and support the immune system

IMMUNOMODULATOR: Balances the immune system, stimulating a suppressed immune system and suppressing an overstimulated immune system

IMMUNOSTIMULANT/IMMUNE STIMULANT: Stimulates the immune system (Also known as *immune stimulant*)

INFUSION: A medicinal remedy made by boiling water, pouring it over herbs, and letting it steep for 1 to 8 hours

INTESTINAL TONIC: Tones the intestines

KIDNEY TONIC: Restores or increases tone in the kidneys

LAXATIVE: Helps produce bowel movements (See also *aperient*)

LITHOTRIPTIC: Dissolves calculi (stones)

LIVER STIMULANT: Stimulates the liver

LIVER TONIC: Restores or increases tone to the liver

LUNG TONIC: Restores or increases tone to the lungs

LYMPHATIC: Cleans and improves lymph flow through the body.

MENSTRUUM: A solvent such as alcohol, glycerin, vinegar, or water that is used to extract constituents from herbs

MOLLUSCIDAL: Kills mollusks (mainly snails and slugs)

MUCILAGINOUS: Contains polysaccharides that create a slippery texture and mild taste with soothing and cooling qualities

MUCOLYTIC: Eases mucus (sputum), making it easier to expel

MUCOSTATIC: Helps stop the secretion of mucus

MUSCLE BUILDING TONIC: Helps build muscle tone

NARCOTIC: Induces a state of stuporous analgesia

NERVE RELAXANT: Relaxes nerves

NERVE RESTORATIVE: Restores nerves

NERVINE: Benefits the nervous system

NUTRITIVE: Nourishes the body

ODONTALGIC: Remedies toothaches

ONEIROGEN: A substance, practice, or experience that promotes or enhances dream states

OPHTHALMIC: Relates to the eye

PARTURIENT: Brings on labor and assists with birth

PECTORAL: Tonifies and strengthens the pulmonary system

PHYTOESTROGENIC: Contains phytoestrogens, plant-based estrogens

POULTICE: A soft, moist mass of herbs that is often heated and applied directly on skin or over a thin cloth to heal and relieve aches and inflammation or reduce pain

PROSTATIC: Supports the prostate

PURGATIVE: A strong laxative

REFRIGERANT: Cools the body from the inside out

REJUVENATIVE: Restores to youthful vigor

RELAXANT: Calms and sooths without sedating

REPRODUCTIVE AMPHOTERIC: Normalizes reproductive function

RESTORATIVE: Returns the body to health

RUBEFACIENT: Herbs for topical application that produce skin redness by dilating capillaries and increasing blood circulation

SALVE: A mixture of oils and a hardening agent such as beeswax to help heal or protect skin

SEDATIVE: Calms, moderates, or tranquilizes nervousness or excitement

SIALAGOGUE: Increases saliva flow

SOPORIFIC: Induces sleep or drowsiness

SPIT POULTICE: Simple poultice made by chewing a fresh leaf and applying it directly to a wound

STIMULANT: Energizes a part of the body

STOMACHIC: Tones the stomach, improving its function and increasing appetite

STYPTIC: Stops bleeding by constricting tissue and blood vessels

SUDORIFIC: Induces sweating

THYROID ENHANCER: Enhances thyroid function

THYROID TONIC: Restores or increases thyroid function

TINCTURE: Preparations made by extracting and preserving the active properties of herbs using alcohol (Also referred to as *extract*)

TISANE: Another name for an herbal tea made by steeping fresh or dried herbs in hot water

TONIC: Restores or increases body tone; also, an herbal preparation, herb, or formula that is taken for an extended period of time to restore or increase body tone

TROPHORESTORATIVE: Nourishes and restores the physiological structure and function of an organ, system, or tissue

URINARY ANTISEPTIC: Prevents urinary tract infection by inhibiting the growth of microorganisms

URINARY TONIC: Tones the urinary tract or increases urinary function

UTERINE DECONGESTANT: Helps remove congestion in the uterus

UTERINE STIMULANT: Energizes the uterus

UTERINE TONIC: Tones the uterus or increases uterine function

VASODILATOR: Widens blood vessels and helps prevent high blood pressure

VASORELAXANT: Causes a decrease in vascular pressure, resulting in reduced tension of blood vessel walls

VERMIFUGE: Expels internal parasites from the body by stunning or killing them without causing significant damage to the host (Also known as *anthelmintic*)

VULNERARY: Helps heal wounds

RESOURCES AND REFERENCES

The following are a few of my favorite herbalism resources. I have included books and publications that are related to herbal healing, as well as websites where you can source everything from herbs and seeds to containers. I've also listed some educational resources to help you further your herbal education.

Books and Magazines

Backyard Medicine, 2nd Edition, by Julie Briton-Seal and Matthew Seal. 2019.
Another great book to help you learn about the plants growing in your own backyard.

The Essential Herbal (essentialherbal.com).
A bimonthly print publication filled with articles about herbs, written by herbalists from around the United States.

The Forager's Harvest (2006) and *Nature's Garden* (2010), by Samuel Thayer.
Both of Samuel's books are great resources for anyone learning to wildcraft. He provides identification, plus the medicinal and edible uses of the plants.

Herbal Healing for Women, by Rosemary Gladstar. 1993.
Everything by Rosemary is a gem! This book is specific to women's health, but I highly recommend all her books.

Herbal Roots zine (www.herbalrootszine.com).
I launched this herbal pdf publication for kids in 2009. There are more than 130 different issues, each focusing on one herb with activities to make learning about herbs fun.

The Male Herbal, 2nd Edition, by James Green. 2007.
There are very few male-centric herbalism resources available. This is one of my all-time favorites that I refer to time and again when working with male clients.

Midwest Foraging, by Lisa M. Rose. 2015.
If you want to get into foraging, Lisa's book is a great one to have on hand.

Naturally Healthy Babies and Children, by Aviva Jill Romm, MD. 2003.
   For babies and children, Aviva's books are a great choice. She has also
   written books about women's health.

Herbs and Supplies

Companion Plants (companionplants.com)
   If you want to grow plants, this is a wonderful place to find bare root plants.

Herbalist & Alchemist (www.herbalist-alchemist.com)
   This is my favorite source for ready-made tinctures for adults and children.

Herb Pharm (www.herb-pharm.com)
   This site offers high-quality liquid herbal products for the whole family.

Mountain Rose Herbs (www.mountainroseherbs.com)
   Mountain Rose Herbs sells a variety of products for herbal medicine
   making: high-quality herbs, oils and butters, containers, seeds, and
   even tinctures and infused oils.

Pacific Botanicals (www.pacificbotanicals.com)
   This is another great source for high-quality herbs.

Strictly Medicinal Seeds (strictlymedicinalseeds.com)
   Richo Cech and his wife offer a huge selection of medicinal herb seeds
   and plants.

The Thyme Garden Herb Co. (www.thymegarden.com)
   This is another great source for seeds and some plants.

Education

There are many great schools and online courses where you can get an
herbal education. The ones below are a few of my favorites. For a longer list of
herbalism schools, check the American Herbalists Guild's website.

Chestnut School of Herbal Medicine (chestnutherbs.com)

Herbal Academy (theherbalacademy.com)

Herbmentor: The Herbal Village and Learning Companion
(learningherbs.com/herbmentor)

Websites

American Botanical Council (abc.herbalgram.org)
   A great resource for learning what's going on in world of herbal medicine.

American Herbalists Guild (www.americanherbalistsguild.com)
   A great educational resource for new and experienced herbalists. You can find a Registered Herbalist in your area if you'd like to work with a professional, herb schools around the country if you are interested in getting a more formal education, and lots of information.

Herbalists Without Borders (hwbglobal.org)
   This nonprofit organization is run by volunteers to bring compassionate holistic care to those facing a natural disaster, violent conflict, poverty, trauma, and other access barriers to health and wellness.

Sustainable Herbs Program (sustainableherbsproject.com)
   Learn more about the sustainable growth and supply of medicinal herbs in the commercial market.

United Plant Savers (www.unitedplantsavers.org)
   Committed to saving endangered herbs that are native to the United States, this organization offers lots of information on how you can help preserve our fragile plants.

References

Culpeper, Nicholas. *Culpeper's Complete Herbal: Over 400 Herbs and Their Uses.* London: Arcturus Publishing Limited, 2016.

Griggs, Barbara. *Green Pharmacy: The History and Evolution of Western Herbal Medicine.* Rochester: Healing Arts Press, 1997.

Strehlow, Wighard and Gottfried Hertzka. *Hildegard of Bingen's Medicine.* Santa Fe: Bear & Company, 1988.

Woodward, Marcus. *Gerard's Herbal: The History of Plants.* Guernsey: The Guernsey Press Co. Ltd., 1994.

GENERAL INDEX